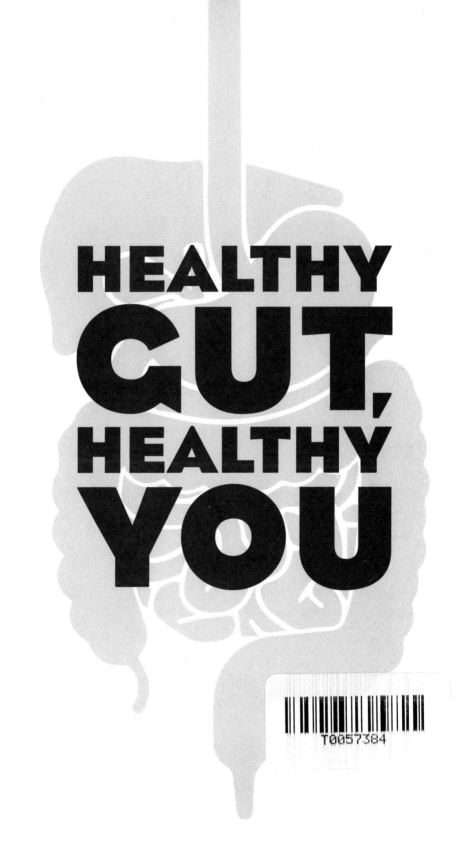

HEALTHY GUT, HEALTHY YOU

The Intestinal Truth

HEALTHY GUT, HEALTHY YOU

Dr. Adrian Schulte

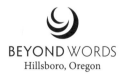

BEYOND WORDS
Hillsboro, Oregon

BEYOND WORDS

8427 N.E. Cornell Road, Suite 500
Hillsboro, Oregon 97124-9808
503-531-8700 / 503-531-8773 fax
www.beyondword.com

First Beyond Words paperback edition February 2019

Copyright translation © 2019 by Beyond Words Publishing, Inc.

Originally published in German (978-3-95803-025-1). Copyright © 2016 Adrian Schulte and
Scorpio Verlag GmbH & Co. KG München.

Managing Editor: Lindsay S. Easterbrooks-Brown
Copyeditor: Gretchen Stelter
Proofreader: Ashley Van Winkle
Design: Devon Smith
Composition: William H. Brunson Typography Services

For more information about special discounts for bulk purchases, please contact Beyond Words
Special Sales at 503-531-8700 or specialsales@beyondwords.com.

Manufactured in the United States of America

10 9 8 7 6 5 4 3 2 1

Library of Congress Cataloging-in-Publication Data

Names: Schulte, Adrian, 1963– author.
Title: Healthy gut, healthy you : the intestinal truth / Dr. Adrian Schulte.
Other titles: Alles Scheisse?! English
Description: First Beyond Words paperback edition. | Hillsboro, Oregon :
  Beyond Words, 2018. | Includes bibliographical references and index.
Identifiers: LCCN 2018040471 | ISBN 9781582706627 (pbk.)
Subjects: LCSH: Gastrointestinal system—Diseases—Alternative
  treatment—Popular works. | Digestion--Popular works. |
  Indigestion—Popular works. | Food—Composition. | Nutrition—Popular
  works. | Self-care, Health—Popular works.
Classification: LCC RC806 .S3813 2018 | DDC 616.3/3—dc23
LC record available at https://lccn.loc.gov/2018040471

The corporate mission of Beyond Words Publishing, Inc.: *Inspire to Integrity*

For Justine, Josephine, Nathan, and Elliott

Contents

PART 3: On the Right Track

Introduction

Are you feeling like crap? We want to feel alive and fresh every day. We want to be healthy and able-bodied and remain young forever, but the reality is that many of us . . . well, we feel like crap.

To do something about it, we focus on living a healthy and sustainable lifestyle, especially when it comes to food. The media is constantly reporting on nutrition. Headlines, trends, and self-help ideas keep popping up everywhere and are either celebrated for a while or ridiculed. But we often forget the most important factor. In your midsection, you carry a powerful organ that makes sure your food is adequately digested and metabolized: the intestines—your second brain.

The organs that make up the intestines are fascinating and, for the most part, work autonomously from the other organs. We should befriend the gut, but too many times, it becomes our enemy. We neglect our bowels and don't know how to treat them well. When we think about how many people suffer from constipation, colon cancer, diverticulitis, intestinal infections, or irritable bowels, one thing is clear—our intestines are not doing well. Twenty years ago, only the elderly suffered from these sicknesses. Today, they affect almost every age group. In recent years, science has shown that a sick bowel can trigger many lifestyle diseases, such as cardiovascular diseases and cancer—even the psyche and spinal cord are affected by the intestines.

But how can we draw any conclusions about our intestinal health when we don't even look at our daily bowel movements to check on the health of our intestines?

It's no wonder so many people are confused. They feel threatened by certain ingredients or intestinal germs and hope that there will be a pill for it one day. But research in this field has proven that our intestinal health, and specifically our intestinal bacteria, depends on what and how we eat. Many nutritional components can harm an already-weakened bowel. But what weakens the bowel? How can we improve its health?

The way we eat has changed as much as our health has over the past one hundred years. I've wondered for a long time now if we haven't forgotten the right way to treat our intestines, putting our health in danger.

I grew up in the sixties, the child of a psychologist and a naturopath. I practically inherited my interest in medicine. At the time, the world was right—at least when it came to food. Vegetables came from your own garden, and there was meat or fish twice a week for lunch. We bought milk from a neighboring farm. My father was the fastest eater I had ever seen. I remember being fascinated with his large stomach. In those days, I didn't think a sick bowel had anything to do with it.

During college and medical school, I lived off of hamburgers and noodles, not only because I didn't know how to cook, but also because fast food was becoming popular. After dissecting a corpse in my first anatomy class, though, I couldn't decipher what kind of meat I was eating in the cafeteria, so I decided to become a vegetarian for almost two years.

After finishing my degree in medicine, I went to London and specialized in tropical diseases. It was then that I discovered that even people in far-off tropical lands were starting to experience lifestyle diseases due to the westernization of their diet. Over the last few thousand years, our intestines have gotten used to a specific feeding pattern, and a rapid change in diet causes diseases. I also learned that these diseases can be controlled by going back to our traditional eating patterns. This caught my attention.

I continued my education in natural medicine and received an offer to take over as medical director of a community health center. It specialized in the regeneration of the intestines. Patients were treated according to a concept by Austrian doctor Franz Xaver Mayr, who focused on the functional improvement of digestive tracts.

It was the first time I realized that our intestines play a crucial role in the state of our health. I witnessed how illnesses improved or disappeared during treatment, even if the issue didn't initially appear to be related to the intestines. Since then, I have gathered twenty years of experience in this field, which I've successfully used to treat patients, and I wrote this book to share that information—the information you need to find your way back to healthy eating habits.

These days, the human digestive tract is overloaded with an endless supply of modified food, whether it's modified by the food industry or genetically. We eat too fast, too much, and too often. We need to remember the basics of a healthy diet, which is more effective than trying one extreme nutritional concept after the other, only to discover that our intestines can't handle it.

Here, you will learn what exactly happens in your stomach and which part of the wonderful digestive process, and your overall health, you can influence in a positive way by simply modifying your eating habits. Everything you experience on the toilet—the color, smell, and consistency of your bowel movement—will tell you if your digestive system is working properly or not.

Very few people need to remove certain foods from their diet entirely. Most of us just have to focus on the quality and amount of food we eat. For example, the right dose of good dairy products is not bad for everyone, just like good bread doesn't make everyone sick.

You are going to learn which diseases are causally related to the intestines, but I'll share more than just what can go wrong; I will show you how easy it is to be in control of your digestion. One way is through your eating habits. Another way is through a ten-day fitness program for your intestines. During my twenty years of experience applying Mayr's concept in diagnosing and treating patients, I have seen excellent results using this fitness program. The intestines can rest and relax, which not only keeps your bowel happy but also helps prevent illness in general.

I'd also like you to eventually be able to decide for yourself which foods are right for you and which ones you need to avoid. It's easy to tell what doesn't sit right, leads to flatulence, or makes your stool smell. (Often, all you need to do is chew more.) To make it easier on you, I evaluate the most common foods based on their digestibility.

You're probably confused about what to eat and what to avoid when you consider all the changes in our eating habits, our modified food supply, and some extremely contradictory recommendations in this area. I'd like to help you find out what is right for your intestines and overall health, and guide you through the hype about your intestines and diet. This book is based on personal experience in my clinic as well as others' scientific discoveries. Since it should be easy to read and relate to, I've tried to avoid citing many references in the text. You can find sources and additional literature in the appendix.

Why the Product
Is So Important

Dookie. Crap. Number two. We have a lot of words for our bowel movements, but honestly, we're normally using them as curses, choosing which to use based on how angry we are or who our audience is. It's a paradox—how many words can we have for a single substance and continue to not actually discuss the substance itself? When the truth is, the many differences that can show in our poop—consistency, frequency, color, smell—are incredibly accurate indications of our health. All we have to do is pay attention.

There are a variety of colors, from light yellow and brown tones to dark brown or even black. The consistency can range from watery, runny, and soft to mushy or hard. As covered on the Bristol Stool Chart, it can come out as thin as a pencil, in little balls like a sheep's, or as a big, fat sausage. It can be, unfortunately, sticky, slimy, bloody, and I'm sure you could think of more, right? But barely anyone thinks about what the consistency means for the organs where our food is processed and that are, therefore, some of the most important organs of all: our intestines.

Our four-legged friends' digestive health receives much more attention than our own. Imagine the following scenario: Man's best friend leaves a pile of loose stool on the sidewalk. All right, you just have to deal with it. So you pull a plastic bag around your hand and try to pick up anything that doesn't ooze out. If it were us, loose or otherwise, we'd just push a button and the problem would be solved. What we wouldn't do to have a button for our best friend's poo too!

In this instance, however, you first look around to see if there are any witnesses and then nonchalantly cross the street. And then? Maybe you make an appointment with the vet. Your pet might have an intestinal inflammation or worms or both—or worse. His coat hasn't been as shiny the past few days. Clearly something is wrong with his food or digestion. But if we were dealing with the same issues, we'd probably focus on the shiny hair and try a new shampoo and be done with it. We wouldn't even consider our digestion.

Now, imagine you're on a walk one day and your poor doogie leaves an extremely stinky pile on the sidewalk—and some on his behind after he's finished with his business. Maybe it leaves a residue that makes people switch sides of the street all afternoon. If you're lucky, you perhaps have your disinfecting spray along and are able to wipe up the rest of the sticky mess, like an upstanding citizen. If it's bad enough, you grab a roll of toilet paper when you get home and rub his bottom clean.

In this case as well, you'd end up in the vet's waiting room a couple of hours later. Not only because you'd get tired of rubbing your dog's butt, but also because you'd want to be sure there is nothing wrong with his bowels.

If you don't take care of it, someone might call an animal welfare agency, because we are responsible for our four-legged friends.

But none of this applies to us. We don't know anything about our intestines and cannot recognize their warning signals. When they're sick, we don't have a clue unless a section gets twisted up and sends us running to the hospital.

ARE YOU UP FOR A LITTLE TOILET HISTORY?

The first flush toilets were patented in the United States in the mid-nineteenth century and soon found their way to Europe via England. It was an invention that practically did away with the possibility of judging the health of our bowels from our bowel movements. Floats or sinks; floats and stinks; sinks and stinks—that was the extent of the information the new type of toilet had to offer. The foul-smelling feces that a sick bowel produces would pass through the air in a fraction of a second before vanishing into the depths. Yet in spite of this very brief "air passage time," new air fresheners, toilet cleaners, and those overpowering little blue blocks were unrelentingly being produced. Why does no one find this odd?

Shelf-style (also sometimes *wash-out* or *shallow flush*) toilets lasted the longest in German-speaking countries. These models are designed with a shelf where the feces can be seen and smelled until they are flushed into the sewage system by a kind of waterfall.

They only exist in German-speaking countries now! You might get some funny looks if you were to order one, but at least they are still being manufactured, as they should be. Not only do they make the daily inspection of color, texture, and smell easier, but also collecting a stool sample for the doctor is a simple matter.

But if the washdown toilet doesn't leave any clues behind, there's another way of finding out about our bowel health: toilet paper. It would be great if we didn't need any. It may not happen often, but we're all familiar with that great feeling we get when the toilet paper stays clean after wiping. The large intestine coats the stool in a layer of mucus, preventing the anus from being soiled—something we take for granted in our four-legged friends.

Each one of us uses an average of thirty-three pounds of toilet paper every year, and we think that's normal. We might sometimes worry about the rain forests, but we certainly don't think about what it says about our own health. In spite of current deep-flush toilets, toilet paper can provide us with important information about the state of our bowels (traces of blood on the paper, for example). However, it may not be around for much longer. Often the only way of thoroughly cleaning the anal area is through sophisticated rinsing and blow-drying techniques, which are beginning to take over the market.

Now for some crucial questions: What should stool from a healthy bowel look like? How should it smell? What consistency should it have?

Many people have no idea; they only look in the toilet bowl when they have to vomit. But it doesn't have to be that way. That is why I am going to tell you what our stool is made of—perhaps a greater understanding will help relieve you of your disgust.

One part consists of food residue that we are unable to digest or break down by bacterial processes in our bowels. A fiber-rich diet increases this part and thus the quantity of stool produced.

It also consists of dried mucous membrane. Just like your skin, your intestinal mucous membrane is constantly renewing itself. The mucous membrane lining your small intestine has a surface area of approximately 3,230 square feet, and it renews itself every two to three days. That means 3,230 square feet of mucous membrane down the toilet every two to three days. That's a lot. If you suffer from enteritis, or intestinal irritation, the quantity of excreted mucous membrane increases, just like the skin on your back renews itself more quickly when your sunburn peels. When that happens, the quantity of stool increases and you have more frequent bowel movements.

Your poo is also made up of bacteria, both dead and alive. If we were to search our surroundings with a microscope, we would discover that bacteria can be found everywhere: tables, chairs, the floor—everywhere. A good third of our digestive waste is made up of bacteria. The colon, which is close to the outer body, promotes the growth of germs and is inhabited by large quantities of bacteria and some fungi.

To sum it up, dead mucous membrane, bacteria, and indigestible food make up the stuff we blindly flush away. There's no reason to be grossed out. As long as our digestion is healthy, it doesn't even stink. It's only when our bowels don't do their job properly that it begins to get disgusting—when processes of fermentation and putrefaction transform our feces into a foul-smelling, sticky, more or less solid mass.

As far as color goes, there's a wide spectrum of healthy variations, depending on what you've been eating. So don't worry! Every shade of brown, green after a meal of spinach, red after beets, or even black after blueberries. But watch out, because green without spinach, red without beets, and black without blueberries can be signs of a serious illness. The use of supplements can also affect the color of your stool; for example, iron supplements create a very dark, black stool.

It's the smell that reveals something isn't right most quickly. Our stool should be almost odorless. If it smells sour, rotten, or fetid, it is unhealthy! The consistency also provides us with clues. Healthy stool is neither very hard and lumpy nor watery or mushy.

Unfortunately, the number of bowel movements is often the only criterion used to measure bowel health. Five times a day is too often; once a week is not enough. Once every morning would be normal. But twice a day is normal, too, if the stool properties named above are normal.

Let's assume for a minute that you have one of these happy bowels. Your bowel movement is regular, your stool is well formed and almost odorless, and the only reason you keep toilet paper around is because the jokes printed on it make you laugh, or you like the flowery pattern. In that case, you can lay this book aside and turn to something more interesting.

Perhaps, though, there is someone in your family or group of friends who is less fortunate and could do with some valuable advice, or you would simply like to know what's going on with that coworker of yours who used the toilet before you a few days ago and left you feeling as if you'd been gassed. In that case, you should continue reading.

The digestion process can be compared to an assembly line—one or more workers work at each stage of digestion, and the stool is the finished product.

If everything is running smoothly in a factory, it shows in the quality of the product. If anything is wrong with the product, you have to take a tour of the factory to find out just where things are being messed up. I'm going to take you on a tour like that. We will find mistakes that are easily fixed and other mistakes that require a medical examination and advice.

To avoid losing track of what's what in the following parts, it helps to take a closer look at the digestive tract one more time:

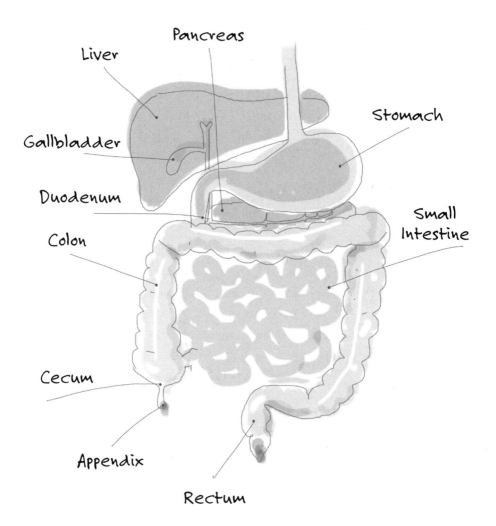

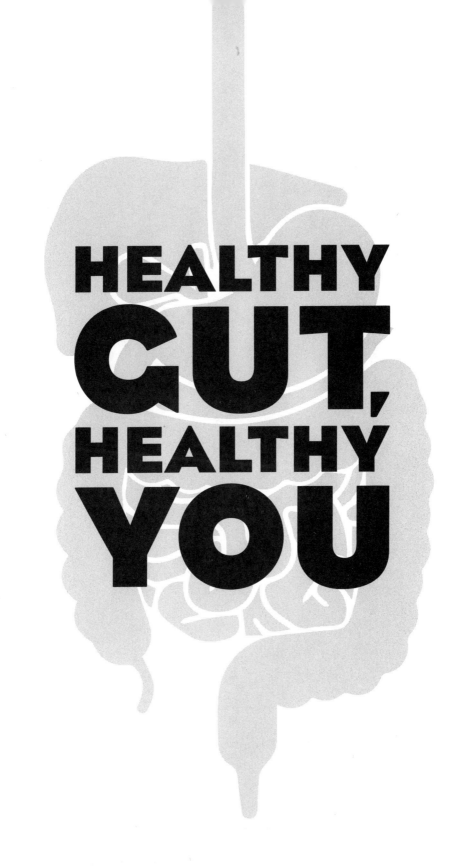

1

A TRAVEL GUIDE TO YOUR DIGESTIVE TRACT

UNTAPPED POSSIBILITIES: SMELLING, TASTING, CHEWING

Our cells consume energy. To provide them with this energy, we have to ingest food. That may not sound too appealing to a gourmet, and it would be a shame if eating was reduced to a purely physical level, but it is basically what drives us.

But how do we figure out what is good for us and what isn't, or what to buy and what's best to avoid? It's our sensory organs that make those decisions for us.

Taste and Smell

In the US and German-speaking countries (societies that have become more commercialized, with packaged foods) we tend to make decisions about what to eat based on what our eyes tell us. While in Mediterranean countries, touch and smell often play a role, since fresh foods are bought in local markets. We buy and eat better-quality fruits and vegetables if we use our sensory organs to provide our control center, the brain, with as much information as possible. In France, this is taught in school. *Classes du goût* are an integral part of their class schedule. Even the youngest pupils learn to train their senses of sight, touch, taste, and smell, so they can buy and enjoy their food with greater awareness. Granted, sniffing and manhandling produce before paying for it wouldn't make you very popular in some places, but it's a good idea all the same. We would discover that tomatoes picked abroad before ripening may have traveled long distances, but they haven't acquired much smell. If we decided to take them home anyway, we would soon discover that they don't have much taste either.

Once the tomatoes have been prepared at home, smell is joined by taste. Ten thousand taste buds, which is more than in any other animal, help us make a correct judgment. A cat, for example, has a mere five hundred. Cats are carnivores. It wouldn't occur to them to eat roots, vegetables, mushrooms, or grains, so they have no need for taste buds that tell them whether those foods are good or bad. But they do have a highly sophisticated and well-trained sense of smell that kicks in even before their sense of taste starts working. If you offer a cat something rotten, it will wrinkle up its nose and walk away. We'd be spared a lot of cases of food poisoning if we used our noses more. Think of the smell of a bad mussel or oyster or rotten meat. Those are difficult smells to forget.

Smell and taste are closely related. You know what it's like when you have a cold and can't smell properly—the things you eat have less taste than usual too. Or try holding your nose while you're eating; you can hardly taste anything.

But how do we get our taste buds to explode like fireworks of flavor? To make full use of our sense of taste, whether for the purpose of choosing food or enjoying it, we must keep the food in our mouths for as long as possible. Swallowing after two bites is not enough to activate our taste buds. But if they are activated, and we like the taste of the food, something amazing happens. The brain pumps out dopamine, serotonin, and naturally produced opioids. These are messengers that leave us feeling not only full but also satisfied after a meal.

Unfortunately, our sense of taste is easily tricked. High-quality, healthy food tastes good. That's how we know we've made the right choice. But food that has lost its taste (if it ever had any in the first place) during the process of industrial production has flavoring or "aromas" added to it.

The food industry has been doing this for decades. The majority of food consumed nowadays would never make it onto our tables if it weren't for these added aromas. If you were to chew this food for a long time, you would notice that, unlike the taste of good-quality, healthy food, the taste provided by the artificial flavoring soon disappears. It is easy to tell the difference between artificially flavored food and fresh, healthy food. Try it yourself sometime!

Our sense of taste does something else too. It triggers digestion. If we taste something sweet, the pancreas is stimulated to produce insulin. We need insulin to process the sugar we eat, but we only want so much insulin, as the fat reserve that some of us would like to get rid of is not broken down when insulin is at work. Fat burning is blocked. It would not be very efficient to break down fat reserves when high-energy sugar is on the way. That is why eating sweet things between meals has a doubly negative effect on our energy balance.

We can assume that other taste sensations stimulate digestion. Let us imagine this scenario: We eat a bowl of yogurt with artificial strawberry aroma. The workers on the digestion assembly line are informed, and they get the tools ready to digest strawberries. But they don't see any of the fruit they were expecting. Unfortunately, we know next to nothing about the consequences of such deception, but it's easy to imagine a bunch of workers standing around with the wrong tools in their hands. They'd probably start losing interest in coming to work. They might even go on strike if we send a real strawberry their way.

Conclusion: Use all the senses at your disposal when choosing food. Eating will be more of a pleasure and your health will benefit too.

Chewing: The key to Healthy Digestion

Chewing is the first step in digestion, and as you will see, it is also the last step you can actively participate in. That is why it is extremely important for us. The digestion that takes place in the mouth primarily consists of producing saliva and chewing.

Saliva can be produced without our involvement as well, like when something makes our mouths water, which can happen even when our mouths are empty. The main control center, your brain, processes information sent to it by your eyes—when you have spotted something tasty—or it processes purely mental information, such as when you imagine something sweet you'd like to eat.

We know of two different kinds of saliva. Watery saliva flows into your mouth like water to counteract something spicy or very sweet. Gel saliva, on the other hand, is produced by active chewing. We need it to lubricate the food we eat. Without it, you would have difficulty getting food down your esophagus. Of course, there is a trick, but it's not good for digestion. You can rinse the unchewed food down with a drink, without having produced the necessary saliva beforehand. But, as you will see later, this takes its toll on your stomach.

Gel saliva also contains an enzyme that begins to digest carbohydrates. That means that the splitting of the long carbohydrate chains that we call *starch* begins in the mouth. You can taste this if you carry out a little experiment. Chew an old piece of bread at least thirty times, and you will notice the pulp in your mouth gradually growing sweet. The short chain sugars that have been enzymatically split taste sweet to us, and the long chain sugars don't.

As we chew, the necessary gel saliva is produced, but there's more. The chewing reduces the food to smaller pieces in order to digest it properly, while activating our sense of taste. An intense taste experience gives us a sense of being full (the sensory-specific satiety), which has nothing to do with a full stomach, and allows us to finish a meal without feeling bloated and tired.

People who chew more consume fewer calories. This was demonstrated in a study that used video cameras to compare the eating habits of slim and overweight men. The overweight men did not take larger bites than the men of normal weight, but they ate more quickly, chewed less, and spent longer eating. The study showed that good chewing reduced calorie intake by an average of 11.9 percent. Assuming the men of normal weight had a daily intake of 2,000 calories, insufficient chewing would mean a calorie intake of approximately 238 calories more. In one year, that would add up to an excess of about 86,870 calories, which corresponds to about twenty-two pounds of fat! Of course, exercise, stress, and many other factors also play a role.

However, why was the calorie intake lower? Thorough chewing leads to less of the appetite-stimulating hormone ghrelin in our blood and a simultaneous increase in the appetite-suppressing hormones glucagon-like peptide-1 and cholecystokinin.

And that's not all. Chewing also improves circulation in the brain and enhances mental performance. Thorough chewing following an intestinal operation speeds up the recovery process. Recurrent bowel obstruction following an intestinal operation can be prevented by vigorous chewing. All of which demonstrates that good chewing has a significant influence on digestion, metabolism, and brain circulation.

So why do we hardly ever see anyone chewing properly? This hasn't always been the case. There's an old German saying, "Proper chewing leads to healthy digestion," and many of us can remember a grandmother telling us to chew each bite thirty-two times. This rule was established by the British politician William Gladstone, who thought we should chew each bite thirty-two times because we have thirty-two teeth. Horace Fletcher demonstrated how chewing can help us maintain or restore our health. Franz Xaver Mayr included chewing training in the treatments he developed to restore the performance of the digestive tract and healed many of his patients that way. How did all this knowledge get lost?

Until the mid-twentieth century, we were expected to do something for our own health. Each individual was partly responsible for his or her health. The simpler the method, the more popular it was. It was an established fact that chewing aided digestion, thereby improving general health. However, such foundations for a healthy life were lost, as our society found itself struggling more and more with excess, and our healthcare system gradually took the burden of responsibility from the individual. Patients started to fill doctors' waiting rooms, and there was a pill for just about everything. The emerging fast-food society replaced traditional eating cultures, and knowledge about the health-preserving qualities of chewing vanished.

The time we set aside for meals grew increasingly shorter. The shorter the meal, the faster, and as a result, the more people ate. Good chewing became almost impossible. The proportion of industrially manufactured meals rose and with it the use of artificial aromas, which were added to compensate for the taste that was lost in the food's production. This has made it difficult for us to return to our former eating cultures. If the aroma vanishes after a couple of chews, we get no pleasure from prolonged chewing and inevitably send the food swiftly on its journey.

Good chewing makes for longer meals, of course. At least, it does if you chew well and slowly. Chewing in slow motion—how annoying. You're still on your first course while everyone else is hitting the dessert. Your friends stop inviting you to their dinner parties. But it is possible to chew well and quickly! You can find training instructions in part 3 of this book.

A good hundred years ago, Horace Fletcher made a name for himself by using exaggerated chewing to improve his health and that of his followers. It's a story that will get your jaw muscles moving.

Horace Fletcher

Chewing guru Horace Fletcher was born in the United States in 1849. He was a very successful entrepreneur. Manufacturing and selling cheese made him rich. At the age of forty, he was five feet six and weighed 217 pounds. His waistline measured sixty-one inches. During fifteen years of highs and lows, he battled with his weight and, increasingly, with his health. Not only did he feel tired, worn out, and weak, but he was also short of breath and suffered from arrhythmias. Gout plagued his joints. He knew he probably didn't have a lot longer to live, so he started to take better care of himself.

"You have to walk more and chew better," recommended a lively older man. It was worth a try, so in mid-June in 1897, he began his experiment. He chewed and insalivated every single bite (admittedly a bit over the top) until there was no taste left and it would slide down his throat without him consciously swallowing.

The results were incredible. In September 1913, he weighed 162 pounds, and his waistline had shrunk by 23.6 inches. During the experiment, he made do with one meal per day (he wanted to lose weight quickly) that consisted of about thirty bites, which he chewed about 2,500 times in total. The meal lasted at least thirty minutes. The dishes were mostly meat and fish with potatoes and vegetables, bread and butter. Between meals, he only drank water.

For a few weeks, he was worried about his digestive tract, which had been worn out through years of abuse. At first, he had irregular bowel movements. But once he became regular again, his stool—or "digestive ash," as he called it—was entirely odorless.

His overall health did a complete 180° within a mere four months. He felt strong and fit. His joints no longer hurt. On some days, he rode his bike for over ninety miles without complaining about being sore or tired afterward. And you can imagine what "pedal machines" were like back then, nothing remotely like bicycles of today.

Horace Fletcher wrote several books on the subject, which were translated into many languages. He traveled to Europe to spread his discoveries. First, the science departments at the University of Venice supported him. Then, the president of the English Physiological Society at the time, Professor Sir Michael Foster, invited him to Cambridge, where he could continue focusing on his theory.

Ultimately, the president of the American Physiological Society, Professor Russell Chittenden, performed tests which revealed that Fletcher's physical and mental performance were on par with twenty-year-old students who worked out.

Followers of his method included Upton Sinclair, Henry James, John Rockefeller, Mark Twain, and many others.

If Horace Fletcher hadn't fallen victim to the Spanish flu epidemic in 1919 at the age of sixty-nine, like twenty to forty million other people, he might have lived until the ripe old age of 110. And maybe his method would have been more widespread throughout the general public and fast food might never have become so popular.

THROUGH THICK AND THIN— THE DIGESTIVE FLOW

Swallow or Gag?

Swallowing is the last step we control before the digestive system takes over. We have no direct influence over what happens between the pharynx and the anus. This means we cannot send direct orders to the stomach— *It looks like I didn't chew well enough and swallowed a little too soon. I know you haven't been feeling very well lately, but do you think you could try to do the teeth's job anyway?* That doesn't work at all, unfortunately.

We normally go into autopilot for swallowing, and to regulate it, we have swallow and gag reflexes.

The swallow reflex is triggered when food pulp touches the wall of the throat. If our teeth crushed the pulp small enough, we swallow unconsciously. Try the following: Place an old piece of bread in your mouth and chew thirty to forty times. Your mouth empties itself without you consciously or actively swallowing.

Now take another bite, chew two times, and try pushing it toward your throat. The pharynx contracts and orders the pieces back into the mouth, where they will be broken down further in preparation for swallowing.

Luckily, we have a gag reflex that protects us from swallowing things that are too big. We can, however, trick that reflex by actively swallowing, which makes sense if we have to swallow a large pill for example. Unfortunately, we also use the active swallowing trick to send poorly chewed food on its way. This only partially works in the case of the bread. You'd have to wash it down with a drink, because not enough saliva can be produced in such a short time. That's why we don't call this *swallowing*, but rather *washing it down* or *choking it down*. It's no wonder the back of the throat wall turns increasingly insensitive. The gag reflex is triggered less, while the digestive tract is burdened more with large, unprepared morsels.

Sometimes, we even start making these mistakes in our first years of life. When an almost-toothless toddler eats a meal that should've been cut into smaller pieces, their body will automatically send the food back up. We regularly observe worried parents struggling at mealtime, shoving the spoonful of food back into their child's mouth. Once the gag reflex tires, the training is deemed successful. From then on, the child can choke down abundant amounts of poorly chewed food, making unreasonable demands on their digestive system for years.

By now you've surely asked yourself the question: Do I swallow my food, choke it down, or just wash it down with a drink?

The Stomach Kneads Everything Down— and Doesn't Want Any Troublemakers

Food passes to the stomach a few seconds after entering the esophagus, which pushes the pulp in a *peristaltic* (a radially symmetrical contraction and relaxation of muscles) wave toward the *cardia* (entrance to the stomach). This peristaltic wave works regardless of the body's position. Whether you're sitting, standing, lying down, or even in a handstand, food pulp reaches your stomach.

Let's imagine this process on fast forward. A small piece of the ring-shaped muscle of your esophagus relaxes and expands, takes the food pulp, and immediately contracts, pushing it a little farther down. The whole elaborate process repeats itself until the pulp reaches the sphincter at the cardia, also called the lower esophageal sphincter, which is where the esophagus opens into the stomach.

If ice-cold water hits this sphincter, it blocks the water's passage to the stomach, and the cold liquid sits in the esophagus for a few seconds. This creates a sensation of pain behind the sternum. Your natural body temperature warms up the liquid, allowing it to slowly enter into the stomach, and the pain subsides. We disrupt this shutter mechanism by drinking ice-cold liquids, consuming many types of alcoholic beverages, eating certain spices, and sometimes just by drinking a cup of coffee. This keeps the sphincter from doing what it's supposed to do.

The sphincter ensures that the hydrochloric acid in the stomach doesn't flow up to the esophagus. If it doesn't do its job, we get heartburn, as the acid is so strong that the esophagus becomes enflamed upon contact. We know when this is happening through a burning or pressing sensation behind the breastbone.

It is, therefore, a good idea to avoid anything that causes heartburn. This can be something different for everyone, from coffee to white wine or even cake. If it keeps happening, the cardia will need a break to regenerate. Antacids can help, or even better, a small stomach fitness program since you'd have no problems if your stomach were in better shape. There will be more details about the program in part 3.

The stomach is supposed to receive the food pulp in a pulpy state, as the name suggests. Then, no matter what we've eaten, the hydrochloric acid can do its thing in half an hour and send the *chyme* (mass of pulpy, acidic, partly digested food) to the checkpoint at the *pylorus* (the stomach's exit into the small intestine), where there is another sphincter, the pyloric sphincter.

When this sphincter is working correctly, it only lets pulp out of the stomach if it's liquid. The individual components of food can be no larger than 0.2 millimeters, or they remain in the stomach until they are. That is what the hydrochloric acid is there for. But it can take a while. For instance, a piece of poorly chewed meat takes eight to ten hours. During this time, it is thoroughly mixed and kneaded.

Lions don't chew well and like to eat meat, as much as seventy-seven pounds at once. However, lions have larger stomachs and don't eat meat three times a day. Once they've swallowed their meal whole, they lie in the shade and let their stomachs go to work. About two or three days later, they set off to find their next prey. (It's a good time to stay far away.)

We, on the other hand, do not wait ten hours for the stomach to finish the teeth's job. We eat again after only three or four hours. The stomach cooperates for a while, but not forever. It gets worn out, just like the sphincter at the pylorus does. It stops waiting for meat to become liquid and lets it pass too soon. Normally, digestive enzymes in the duodenum (the first section of the small intestine) have it easy if the meat leaves the stomach in a liquid state. The small intestine absorbs the meat entirely, because it doesn't contain any fiber. This leaves the empty-handed bacteria in the large intestine longing for sustenance.

If, however, the bacteria in the colon come across largish chunks of meat, healthy digestion cannot be guaranteed. If the meat is still on the larger side, it means the small intestine is only beginning the digestion process, not actually digesting. Since the journey through the large intestine takes a long time and the bacterial colony there is so large, it's no wonder that bacteria specializing in putrefaction happily begin to decompose the partially digested chunks of meat.

But let's go back to the stomach for a minute. Improper chewing is not the only thing that makes the stomach work harder. When its hydrochloride acid is in the middle of breaking down food, a flood of cold, fizzy liquid can completely interfere with the process. If the drink is room temperature and not fizzy, it flows past the food pulp without disrupting it, right into the next part, the duodenum. Unfortunately, drinks are typically cold and often fizzy.

Even when the inspector (sphincter) at the stomach's exit (pylorus) is tired and not capable of much more, it won't let cold or fizzy liquids pass through. All the liquid is added back into the gastric acid and food pulp mixture. This leads to a ruckus in your stomach, and digestion takes a lot longer.

Go ahead and try it out for yourself. Drink a glass of cold and really fizzy water or a soft drink on an empty stomach. If the liquid were to pass straight through your stomach, the released gas would blow up the small intestine like a balloon. Luckily, that's not how it works. The fizzy drink stays in the stomach at first. The released gas lingers below your diaphragm, which is a breathing muscle and the divider between the chest and abdominal cavities. This gas bubble makes breathing more difficult, but after one or two strong belches, there is room again for another few sips. It's not easy to drink a lot without straining our stomachs. Therefore, a little effervescence is really nice, but everything else is just torture for the stomach.

The Chinese have known this a long time and tend to drink tea with their meals. In Europe, they sometimes drink red wine or a glass of uncarbonated water, neither of which are cold or fizzy, so it is possible to enjoy a meal without cold and carbonated liquids.

Besides poorly chewed food and cold, fizzy drinks, the stomach has trouble dealing with concentrated grease or oil. If really greasy food reaches the sensory cells at the pylorus, they immediately check the amount of bile present in the gallbladder.

Bile is necessary to digest grease. If there's not enough bile, the stomach stops kneading. This can take anywhere from one to two hours, during which time we do not feel our best, as if we were stuffed, and our breathing becomes shallow and difficult from the pressure under the diaphragm.

People in Normandy, France, made a clever little ritual called *trou normand* to get out of this irritation. It's schnapps to the rescue! And it really does rescue the stomach. They drink a glass of schnapps after the first course to make room for the next course. Within a second of ingesting it, the stomach contracts, and they can breathe again. Sometimes they even feel like eating again.

But the schnapps doesn't trigger digestion, because distilled alcohol isn't able to do that. What it does is irritate the entrance of the stomach (cardia), causing the stomach to instantly contract. This creates space in the upper part of the stomach, but it turns out to be serious torture for the stomach. It's similar to forcing a tired donkey through endless steppes: it walks a lot without getting stronger. And people in Normandy have more cases of cancer of the esophagus than all other Europeans too. It usually originates near the cardia, probably due to excessive irritation of the area. Maybe it's true what they say: everything in moderation.

Fermented alcohol such as wine or beer does actually stimulate the digestive glands. Sadly for some, it also triggers an appetite. One study showed that we eat up to 15 percent more when we drink wine or beer.

Similar to most human organs, the stomach prefers certain times of the day to work. In traditional Chinese medicine, they have assumed for thousands of years that the right time for digestion is in the morning. In the western world, there is a saying for this: "Eat breakfast like a king, lunch like a prince, and dinner like a pauper." In Russia, the saying goes, "Eat breakfast yourself, share lunch with a friend, and give dinner away to your enemy."

If we look at the digestive process under a microscope, we'd realize that the stomach becomes tired in the evening. If we shove it full of food right before going to bed, it won't be happy, making it more difficult for us to breathe and causing restless nights. Unfavorable air pressure is already conducive to snoring; add a little alcohol to the mix, and we have a nighttime symphony. If we want to sleep well at night, all we have to do is eat less dinner.

The stomach is the second workstation on our digestive assembly line. The first workstation consists of teeth. When the first workstation goes on vacation and leaves a lazy, barebones emergency team behind, poorly chewed food arrives in the stomach. The second workstation tries to make up for the missing work from the first station. It works for a while, but the stomach gets tired and overstrained. Cold, fizzy drinks and large dinners make its life even more difficult. The second station soon tires from all the extra work and our basis for good digestion disappears.

It's actually not that difficult to treat our helpful and smart employees well. We can reduce the amount of work they have to perform by ending a meal before we are completely stuffed. Our employees equally love a small dinner and well-chewed nourishment and are eternally grateful if we avoid cold, fizzy drinks during or after meals. This is how our stomachs can prepare our meals for healthy digestion.

The Twelve-Finger-Long Acid Buffer

The duodenum, originating from a Greek word that means "twelve fingers long," is the first section of the small intestine. Since it performs different tasks than the rest of the small intestine, I'll treat it like a separate section. A sealing mechanism separates the duodenum from the stomach to prevent the strong gastric acid from leaking in and causing burns or sores. A few inches from the stomach's exit (pylorus), there is a small hole in the duodenum covered with a sphincter: the major duodenal papilla. It was first illustrated by Gottfried Bidloo in 1685, although it is sometimes called the *papilla of Vater*, after German anatomist Abraham Vater.

That is where the bile duct and duct of the pancreas enter. The strong alkaline and enzyme-rich secretions of these two large digestive glands are added to the chyme (food pulp) at this point. There are two reasons why this is very important. First, the acidic chyme coming from the stomach has to be neutralized immediately by the alkaline liquids, to prevent acid burns. Second, incoming digestive enzymes only work in alkaline environments.

Bile secretion is crucial for digesting grease, and through important enzymes, the pancreas further breaks down nutrients, especially proteins. Enzymes, also called *ferments*, are like effective metabolism workers with a degree in biochemistry. These little guys are highly complex, and chemists understand them far better than I, but what is important to know is that they are necessary to break down nutrients into their smallest components for digestion.

The sensory cells at the pylorus transmit how much of the different juices from the gallbladder and pancreas are needed. If we eat extremely greasy food, the gallbladder sends up to a liter of bile per day. If we eat a lot of protein, the pancreas sends up to two liters of secretion.

Dinner can be a problem when it comes to these secretions. When we are tired and worn out, our bodies don't send enough of these juices, which makes good digestion difficult. The reduced transport and insufficient neutralization of the chyme in the small intestine lead to fermentation if it's fermentable food, like fruit. We may notice this phenomenon in the mornings, when our stomachs aren't flat, but rather large and blown up from the resulting gases.

The Small Intestine

With the longest intestinal section and the largest surface area, the small intestine, where 80 percent of the immune system resides, is a section of superlatives. Without it, we are incapable of living. It is about twenty-three feet long, and chyme takes about two hours to pass through it, which is about as fast as a garden snail. During these two hours, the now-liquid chyme is spread out over twenty-three feet and vital work is performed on a surface area of 3,230 square feet. Yes, 3,230 square feet—more room than most of us have in our entire homes! How can a twenty-three-foot-long, approximately one-inch-thick tube make 3,230 square feet?

The small intestine is the wrinkliest object you can imagine. If we look at these wrinkles under a magnifying glass, we see fingerlike protuberances called *villi*. And if we observe these under a microscope, we'd be surprised to see there are more. On these villi, we find even smaller villi. And if we were to put each and every one of these cells under an electron microscope, we'd discover that every individual cell has brushlike protrusions called *microvilli*. So, microvilli on villi on villi on wrinkles, and soon we have our 3,230-square-foot surface area!

The chyme is usually in a liquid state in the small intestine. This is the only way a two-hour transit time is long enough to break down everything and supply our bodies with the resulting components. To accomplish this, the small intestine swings back and forth without us noticing. It kneads a little, like the stomach, and pushes the ever-decreasing amount of chyme a little farther, in the form of a progressive, wavelike contraction, like the motion in the esophagus mentioned earlier.

All intestinal villi have a blood vessel, so they act as gatekeepers, checking what goes inside us and verifying that the chyme is already small enough to enter. Everything the blood absorbs gets sent to the liver, which acts as a treatment plant and detoxifies anything that earlier filters didn't catch. Afterward, nutrients are sent throughout the body in the blood and are available for all our cells.

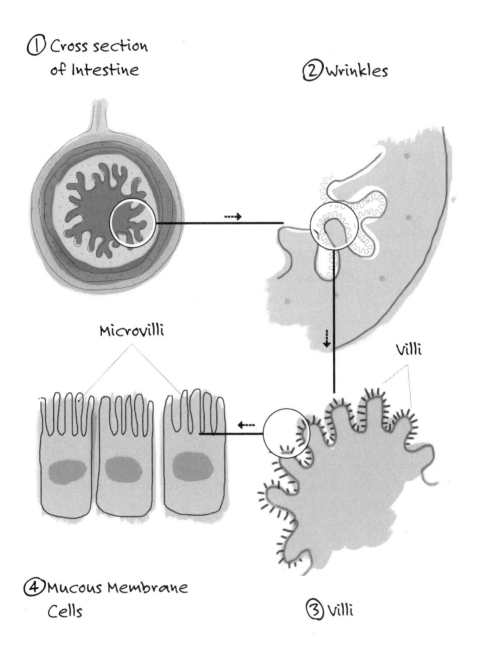

① Cross section of Intestine

②Wrinkles

Microvilli

Villi

④Mucous Membrane Cells

③ Villi

Typically, there are very few bacteria in the small intestine, because the hydrochloric acid in the stomach kills them. If poor chewing or a weak stomach allows a few of them to sneak through, they become victims of a huge cleansing process that is linked to every digestion. The small intestine produces three liters of intestinal juice for this daily cleanse. Just four hours after finishing a meal, the small intestine looks like nothing happened. Shiny, happy villi sit around waiting for their next deployment.

If we can wrap our minds around the entire process (at least two hours to digest and two hours to rest and cleanse), we can clearly see why it is a good idea to wait four hours before eating again. If the cleansing process is interrupted, stray bacteria won't get washed away, and our small intestine gets tired. A sick small intestine can no longer confidently decide what it should absorb, keep for later, or eliminate. Many small meals are not the only things that upset the small intestine though.

After our food (proteins, carbohydrates, and fats) is enzymatically broken down into its smallest components, the mucous membrane absorbs it. Viruses, bacteria, or fungi, along with their metabolites, can sneak up from a densely populated large intestine and interrupt that happy transfer of nutrients. If the mucosa is damaged, more harmful substances can enter the blood, such as very large molecules that should've been broken down earlier, or even bacterial toxins. Our immune cells then react to this "blood poisoning" by releasing inflammatory substances throughout the body that also affect the liver and pancreas. (The exact process is still being researched.)

Sometimes, certain foods trigger this process unexpectedly. Gluten from wheat, for instance, is problematic for some people. It can cause celiac disease, where an immune response damages the villi little by little. This results in the small intestine no longer supplying us with everything that makes us healthy and well nourished.

If an intestinal obstruction interrupts the digestive process, all hell breaks loose within an hour. An intestinal obstruction can be caused by a tumor, hernia (when the intestine gets wedged into a gap in the muscle), or even adhesions, which are basically internal scar tissue from operations. If the flow is interrupted, putrefaction spreads like wildfire, making an intestinal obstruction a true medical emergency.

Additionally, if the chyme arrives in a poorly prepared state or micro-organisms attack, it's not the small intestine's fault that it can't finish digesting within the given time. Because of the extra work and constant overtime, the "workers" don't get enough sleep. You end up getting sick, and in the long run, your body can't withstand the strain.

Shut Your Valve

Located where the small intestine leads into the large intestine is a valve that prevents feces, gases, and bacteria from flowing back into the small intestine from the large intestine. It is called the *ileocecal valve* (ICV) or *Bauhin's valve*. This valve is shut tight and normally only lets digestive leftovers from the small intestine into the large intestine. There is no going back, and that's a good thing. Excessive gas or inflammatory changes in the large intestine can cause the valve to remain partly open, and that has far-reaching consequences.

Toxins originating from bacterial processes in the large intestine are absorbed in much larger quantities in the small intestine, because it is programed to absorb, not fight off toxins. That is why the valve plays such an important role. As long as it remains closed, we're well protected against toxin attacks.

The Large Intestine

There are two reasons to accuse the large intestine of being a slacker.

First, with a transit time of fifteen hours, it's not the fastest. It often loses elasticity over the years and becomes even slower. And second, bacterial putrefaction, fermentation, and all the resulting gases are hard on it.

Even four hundred years before Christ was born, Hippocrates, the founder of Greek medicine and probably the most significant doctor of ancient times, said, "Death sits in the bowels." And the saying, "All diseases begin in the gut" is also from him. He was primarily speaking about the large intestine with that latter quote.

In the United States, somewhere between twenty-five and forty million people suffer from IBS. There are more than 11.6 million cases of appendicitis, an inflammatory condition of the appendix. Approximately one-third of the population older than forty-five and up to two-thirds of the population older than eighty-five suffers from diverticulosis. Additionally, 50 percent of adults have sought out treatment for their hemorrhoids by the age of fifty, resulting in about 20 percent of those cases seeking surgery. More than ninety-five thousand people are diagnosed annually with colon cancer and over fifty thousand will die from it. According to recent research, our intestinal bacteria produce toxins that can make us depressed and other toxins that promote calcification of the arteries and faster aging. Those are enough reasons to take a closer look at this organ.

The predominant environment in the large intestine is an intriguing one. Worms feel especially comfortable there, and there are fifteen thousand times more bacteria in the large intestine than there are humans on earth.

The tasks of the large intestine are clearly defined. One of them consists of absorbing 1.5 liters (50 ounces) of water from the indigestible pulp it receives from the small intestine. This is practical for us, because if it didn't, we'd have to drink this additional amount of water. The large intestine's walls thicken after absorbing water, which explains why it's called the *large intestine*, as it's just a bit larger than the much longer small intestine.

The large intestine's location in the abdomen is precise. It begins on the right side of the lower stomach and leads up, under the right rib cage (the *ascending colon*), where ligaments hold it in place. The transverse colon is the middle part of the large intestine, passing across the abdomen from right to left, below the stomach; the intestine is attached again to the left rib cage. It then heads down, toward the left side of the lower stomach (the *descending colon*), where it makes a slight curve like an *S* on the way outside (*pelvic colon*).

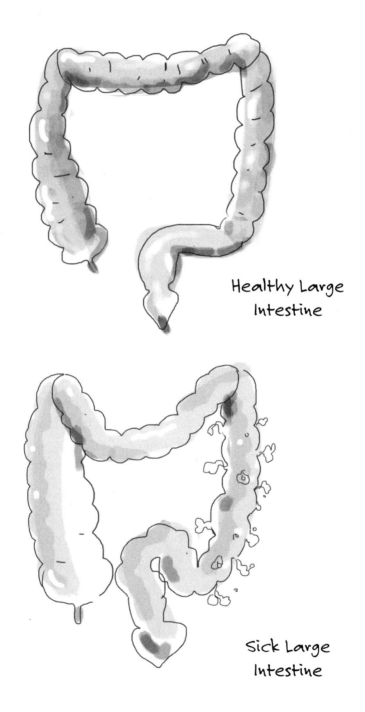

Healthy Large
Intestine

Sick Large
Intestine

It's rather convenient having the intestine attached under the rib cage. It creates an upside-down *U* that in no way blocks the transit of increasingly solid stool. The problem is when the bowel loses elasticity over the years and the transverse colon starts hanging in the middle. It becomes what we call a *sagging colon*. The upside-down *U* becomes a large *M* and the emerging kinks where it's attached under the ribcage become an obstacle for the passing stool (see figure on page 22).

This often leads to constipation that manifests itself in different ways. Sometimes the stool isn't eliminated daily, and when it does pass two or more days later, it's lumpy and solid since a lot of water has been removed.

But why does the big guy lose its elasticity in the first place? As you already know, the entire large intestine has a massive population of bacteria. Anything that is not digested properly along the way falls victim to the bacterial processes in the bowel. It rots or ferments and then lets off gases that we've all smelled before. And if we look closely, we can sometimes recognize what we ate, such as tiny pieces of meat, carrots, or salad.

You may have already witnessed what happens when your intestines get sick. In extreme cases, you can recognize almost everything you ate in your stool. This happens when the passage time through the small and large intestines is greatly reduced. During a normal passage time, the undigested food is broken down by the bacteria in the large intestine. The partially digested meat rots, while the partially digested fruit ferments. During these processes, certain toxins are released that can cause cancer or infections, and they also help us explain the loss of elasticity.

The large intestine reacts to this kind of chemical irritation by mobilizing all its parts to minimize the irritants. It produces more secretion to reduce the concentration of toxins. Additionally, contracting movements send the toxins on their way as soon as possible. And it sends us pain signals, so we know something is wrong. But once a large intestine tires, this defense mechanism is broken and we feel nothing. A stench on the toilet is often the only warning to tell us something is not right. Basically, our large intestine is a kitchen for toxins, and that's everyday life for most people, nothing out of the ordinary.

If we enter large intestine territory, we'll notice that all the wrinkles and villi that we saw in its little brother are missing. Everything looks like large church domes.

The small intestine doesn't lead into the large one by simply becoming larger. It merges sideways into the large intestine, creating about an inch-long pouch called the cecum. (Turn back to page xviii for a diagram.) At the very end of this sack-like section, we find a small, delicate structure that reminds us of an appendage: the appendix. The passage time through the cecum is the second longest in the entire digestive tract (the longest belonging to the rectum). Six hours is considered normal. That is plenty of time for hungry bacteria to gobble up the poorly digested leftovers.

These bacterial processes often lead to inflammation during our childhood years, commonly known as *appendicitis*. When this happens, the delicate appendix is removed to prevent it from bursting, in case it gets too inflamed. All the bacteria from a burst appendix would end up in the abdomen and lead to serious infections.

If the entire cecum is inflamed it's called *typhlitis*. Up until twenty years ago, anyone with pain in this region would instantly be sent to the operating room because of the potential danger. The diagnosis was based on infected cells in the blood, temperatures taken in the armpit and anus, and pressure pain in certain areas of the abdomen. Surgeons tried to base their decision to operate on facial expressions caused by pain, or on the pressure pain threshold in certain postures. Eventually, there was a long list of diagnostic clues. Nevertheless, the pain oftentimes derived from a couple of inflamed lymph nodes in the area. Since the diagnoses were sometimes erroneous, new signs of pain would be checked and added to the long list.

These days, things have changed thanks to the ultrasound. An image of the region allows doctors to see clearly if the appendix is inflamed or not. Consequently, the number of unnecessary appendectomies has decreased. Regardless, around three hundred thousand people undergo appendectomies each year in the United States. The appendix is still keeping surgeons very busy.

The question remains: What else does the appendix do? For a long time, people thought it was a rudimentary organ. This means that it played an important role at one point in human history, yet over time, it started to shrink because we didn't need it anymore. Later, it was discovered to have lymphatic tissue, like tonsils. Located in the digestive tract, where the really long passage time allows for a lot of very nasty bacteria to reside, this lymphatic tissue helps defend against them. A new hypothesis from a research group at Duke University posits that beneficial bacteria that are able, for example, to replenish the bowel after a strong case of diarrhea may also hide here.

Due to the long passage times, 30 percent of malignant colon tumors originate in the appendix area. The other 70 percent develop in the rectum, the last section of the large intestine, where the passage times can be a lot longer.

Where to Next?

The increasingly thick stool is occasionally pushed a little farther by peristaltic movements. After passing the ascending colon and the transverse colon (which is hopefully not sagging yet), feces enter the descending colon, the kingdom of the evil *diverticula*, which are abnormal sacs in the mucosa.

This is where the line starts for the path to the outside, and passage times are especially long. Bacteria and toxins irritate this section of the bowel, producing cramps and contractions so strong that they squeeze the intestinal mucous membrane through the muscle layers of the colon. This is how diverticula emerge, which, as you are about to discover, can cause a lot of trouble.

The formation of a diverticulum can be compared to squishing Play-Doh through your fingers. Your hands represent the intestinal muscles, and the Play-Doh is the solid or gaseous contents of the intestine that get squeezed through your muscles to form the diverticula. They are hollow little pouches where food gets stuck, which can lead to infection. If there are many diverticula, the inside of the bowel looks like swiss cheese. Antibiotics are often used to treat the infection, and if it keeps happening, surgery is required.

The diverticula-infested part of the large intestine is removed to prevent a diverticulum from bursting in the future. Exactly like the appendix, if the bacteria and toxins enter the abdomen, it can lead to a life-threatening infection. In Europe, Australia, and North America, diverticula form in 50 percent of people over sixty. Of these, every fourth person will suffer from one or more infected diverticula in his or her lifetime. In developing countries, where the Western style of eating hasn't been taken up, only 0.5 percent of people over sixty carry diverticula. Infected diverticula and surgery to treat their existence are not at all common in these countries.

The fiber-rich diets in these countries is the reason for this difference. Eating a diet rich in fiber leads to a bowel passage time that's twice as fast, thus lessening putrefaction and fermentation in the intestines. In comparison, the Western diet typically includes a lot of fast food and poorly chewed, low-fiber produce with a high proportion of animal protein and carbohydrates that can't be completely digested in those quantities. Consequently, our bacteria produce a toxic, gaseous concoction that greatly increases the chance of diverticula formation.

When we talk about an irritable colon, we are referring to exactly this region of the large intestine. With so many toxins flying by, it's hard to pinpoint where the irritant comes from.

The next section of the bowel is called the *sigmoid colon (pelvic colon)*. It is the part of the large intestine that is closest to the rectum; it forms a backward *S* on the left side of the lower abdomen. The sigmoid colon is responsible for refilling the rectum once it empties its contents.

The rectum is attached to the sigmoid and ends in an expanded section called the *rectal ampulla*. This is where stool is stored before being eliminated. Malignant illnesses are common in this area due to longer periods of contact with toxic feces, but as long as our digestion is healthy, feces aren't toxic, and cancer is uncommon in this section.

The last part of the large intestine is called the *anal canal*. It is surrounded by two sphincters, but they are not able to completely close the anus. Even when the two muscles contract together, there is still a small opening about one centimeter wide. To save us from having to wear a diaper, there is another muscle along the anal canal plus vascular structures, such as hemorrhoids and vascular cushions, that close the rest of the opening.

We all have hemorrhoids, and in their healthy state, they help us with stool control in the anus. Nevertheless, we only talk about hemorrhoids when the vessels become swollen or inflamed and cause us problems. Those problems arise when blood in these vessels cannot flow properly and the vessel walls are too thin.

There are several possible explanations as to why the blood flow can end up being blocked: large amounts of hard stool, an inflamed anal mucosa, an abdomen overinflated with gases, but also pregnancy or frequent straining for long periods of time.

Which brings us to an interesting subject: toilet behavior. Chronic, frequent straining is often a result of poor posture when going to the bathroom. When we sit or stand, a muscle surrounding our rectum pulls the colon to one side. It's an additional layer of protection to keep us from involuntarily emptying our bowels. Some of my peers actually squat on the toilet seat to achieve the posture that humans have used for thousands of years, because there were no toilets until the eighteenth century. This idea is more for athletic toilet goers, since it requires a certain amount of flexibility and balance. Our intestines would actually be better off if we finally decided to switch our toilets for the Asian squat ones!

However, it's easier to just bend forward. Placing your feet on a footstool like the Squatty Potty can also help. The bowel movement is more complete this way, you don't need to bear down as much, and you only need a third of the time, so you can quickly get back to doing other important things.

In countries where people squat to empty their bowels, they've seldom even heard of diverticula and hemorrhoids. Of course, their diet and eating behaviors are also different—the kind of toilet we use is not the only deciding factor.

When it comes to bowel movements, our intestines have preferred working hours; most people go to the bathroom in the morning, either before breakfast, or after a stimulating cup of coffee. If we ignore this window of time because we have better things to do, we can observe how the bowel is offended and retreats until the next morning. If this happens continuously, it feels like we are no longer taking it seriously and refuses to do its job. Constipation may set in. Furthermore, bacteria have a lot more time to waste and pollute us with toxins. What must come out, must come out. Our bowels have priority.

The workers in these sections of our assembly line suffer. They are sick—not because they make mistakes, but because of prior sloppy work. We sent them too much and too often poorly ground up material.

WHAT COMES IN MUST COME OUT— QUALITY CONTROL

The Little Asshole

The anus, or asshole, is the last section of our entire digestive process that we regulate of our own volition. Thank goodness! Imagine if the large intestine believed it was time to eliminate the finished product while we were eating or at work. Yes, it's a huge advantage to be able to veto bodily functions.

We all know a lot of little assholes—and some big assholes. Why exactly this body part became an offensive swear word is not quite clear, as we should all be elated that we have one and even happier when it works well. But nobody wants to be one. If the anus didn't let off strong-smelling gases and presented a perfectly odorless product each day, the asshole would be as honorable as other body parts, like the ears or nostrils. If we knew at what point *asshole* became a swear word, we might be able to conclude when the health of our intestines started to change. It seems the word first appeared in the Middle Ages.

Could it be that something has been wrong with our digestion for five hundred to a thousand years?

The Product

We can tell by the final product if everything went well during production or if mistakes were made. It's like if you were to park your new car in front of the garage and realize that it had four rearview mirrors, the doors were mounted inside out, the trunk lid was missing, and it had no brakes—you'd be pretty sure that something went wrong in the factory. But if you didn't know what it was supposed to look like, you'd probably be fine with the four rearview mirrors.

It's the same with our stool, only no one told us until now what it's supposed to look like. Because of the market-leading washdown toilets, it's hard to judge if our stool is healthy. It splashes into the water, floats or sinks, and stinks or doesn't. We can usually discern the color, too, as long as floating toilet paper doesn't cover everything.

Many people think that the frequency of their bowel movements is the only indicator of good digestion. As long as they go every day, they assume their digestion is okay without giving it a second thought. But all sorts of sick bowels manufacture an awful product daily, and no one complains because they simply don't know better.

So here are some facts worth knowing about one of the few products that leaves our bodies.

The ideal stool is medium brown, well formed, barely smells, and is covered in a layer of mucus from the intestinal mucosa to prevent the anus from getting dirty on its way out. We wouldn't need toilet paper unless we wanted to be amazed that we didn't need any. We've all experienced this and somehow felt good about it. Some reports mention feelings of bliss—that's how easily amused we can be. The more toilet paper we use, the unhappier we should be, and that includes our intestines.

Daily bowel movements are far from equaling healthy bowel movements. It's important to look closely at frequency and consistency. What does it mean if we go three times a day and the stool looks like porridge?

It could be due to some evil intestinal germs or because we can't digest certain sugars well, like fructose (fruit sugar) or lactose (milk sugar). These sugars ferment in the large intestine and irritate the bowel so much that it has difficulty thickening the stool. It wants to get rid of the product faster and usually more frequently. Or the large intestine becomes so sick over the years that it can no longer thicken properly. Then we also end up disposing of mushy stool several times a day. And the list goes on with possible explanations.

What if we only have one or two bowel movements a week? It means we're constipated, and I'm pretty sure no one mentioned anything about it being blissful. If you can't go every day, it's no big deal as long as the stool doesn't smell. But if it emits a strong, for example rotten, smell, it's a sign you need to free your bowels of the stool every day, and not every other day. A lot of liquids and dried fruits can lend a hand for a while, until you've revved up your intestines again with my fitness program.

Odor is another important signal that everything is running right on the assembly line. This includes any flatulence. During digestion, no gases or odors are produced. Odors and gases only develop later, through bacterial processes in the large intestine, and are either acceptable or problematic. Unpleasant smells are problematic. If your car had an unpleasant smell, you'd ask yourself if everything was okay and what was causing it. The same holds true for smells that are a byproduct of bacterial processes, otherwise known as having gas. If the gas smells rotten, the putrefaction bacteria are active. If it doesn't stink, fermentation bacteria are at work.

Our stool can be a wide spectrum of colors; it depends on what we eat. Everything from light to dark brown is considered normal. If it's especially light, there may be a problem with your bile's flow or production. When it's black, you may need to run to the doctor. If the stool is black and you've not eaten anything that would color it this way, bleeding in the upper digestive tract, such as in the stomach or duodenum, is making it that color. Although the black color could also come from taking charcoal pills or iron supplements.

YOU CAN DO THIS FOR YOUR INTESTINES...

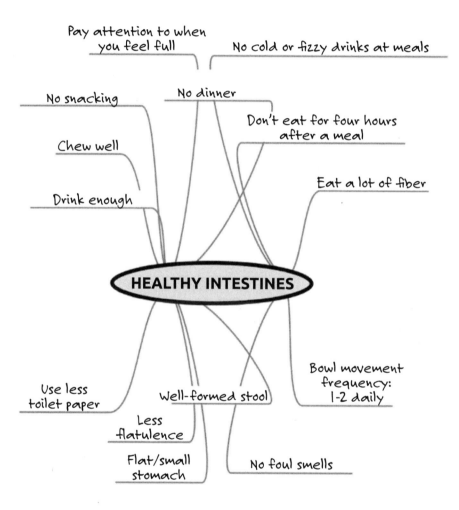

Pay attention to when you feel full

No cold or fizzy drinks at meals

No snacking

No dinner

Don't eat for four hours after a meal

Chew well

Drink enough

Eat a lot of fiber

HEALTHY INTESTINES

Use less toilet paper

Well-formed stool

Bowl movement frequency: 1-2 daily

Less flatulence

Flat/small stomach

No foul smells

...AND THIS IS HOW YOU KNOW THAT EVERYTHING IS GOING WELL!

Red or bloody specks could come from bleeding in the large intestine. Hemorrhoids can announce their presence this way as well. And if we eat red beets, our stool will also turn red—of course, if that's the case, there's no need to worry.

Talking about red beets, they are a good way of showing us how long our intestinal passage time is. If we eat them for lunch, the color normally appears the next morning. Those who don't like red beets can try it with spinach. We can detect worn-out intestines if not only our morning stool is green, but the next day's, stool is, too, and maybe even the day after next. It's a sign that our bowels have become lazy and that we haven't taken self-cleansing very seriously.

The test works with chili as well. Chili should burn twice—one time in your mouth and one time in your anus. This time you don't even need to look in the toilet bowl. If the bowel is tired and the chili has been underway for several days, it doesn't burn the second time around. That's when you know that you have lazy workers down there.

Another way of evaluating passage time and consistency is by using the Bristol Stool Chart, a table that divides the stool into seven different types. It covers all consistencies and shapes: small, hard lumps; lumpy and sausage-like; sausage shaped with cracks; a soft sausage; soft blobs; mushy with ragged edges; and finally, liquid with no solid pieces.

Bristol Stool Chart

Type 1	Separate hard lumps, like nuts (hard to pass)	severe constipation
Type 2	Sausage shaped but lumpy	mild constipation
Type 3	Like a sausage but with cracks on its surface	normal
Type 4	Like a sausage or snake, smooth and soft	normal

Type 5	Soft blobs with clear-cut edges (easy to pass)	mild diarrhea
Type 6	Fluffy pieces with ragged edges, a mushy stool	mild diarrhea
Type 7	Water, no solid pieces, entirely liquid	severe diarrhea

Of course, someone who only has one bowel movement a week doesn't necessarily need the Bristol Stool Chart to know they're constipated. It does help, though, for those who have a lumpy, hard bowel movement every day. They can learn from the chart that something isn't right with their digestion time.

Who would've thought that we could gain insight into how our assembly line is working based solely on the product? Like everything in life, the product that comes out is important. Why shouldn't it be true in this case? But the question remains as to what we need to do to be able to see an excellent product in the toilet and, in many respects, benefit from it.

Quality Management

Do you feel up to a little quality management? Let's go over it all one more time: Digestion starts in your mouth. Then the food is transported down the esophagus to the stomach, by swallowing, and from there, it's sent to the duodenum through the checkpoints of the stomach. After that, it's on to the small intestine, which swings sideways into the beginning of the large intestine, creating a blind-ended tube—the cecum. The large intestine is the last section, where the leftovers are sent out in a bowel movement through the anus into your toilet bowl. This entire process takes about eighteen hours.

Here's something that might be new to you: All these sections are connected by nerve pathways, so every worker on the assembly line knows if everyone is at their station and if they're working hard or may be sick. Most of them work autonomously and don't depend on orders from above—the brain. Our muscles, for example, can't do anything without the brain. If the brain shuts down, everything shuts down. But it's a completely different case for our intestines.

When necessary, the CEO (our brain) gets involved to help regulate things. But we can only influence our completely unconscious processes indirectly, through our actions. This isn't difficult, and it's very effective!

It's unbelievable how easy it is. You'll inevitably ask yourself if it's really possible to influence your bowel health, and thus your health in general, by chewing thoroughly, avoiding snacks, and eating smaller meals.

Yes, it's not only possible, but it's also the only way! If you manage the quality of your intestines, you will notice that you feel good, or at least better, and you can evaluate daily if your bowel is doing a good job based on the product—your feces. Of course, specific intestinal diseases require specific treatments and a mandatory visit to your doctor.

Now that you have extensive knowledge about your digestive process, you can finally take the necessary—maybe even long-overdue—steps to change your eating behavior.

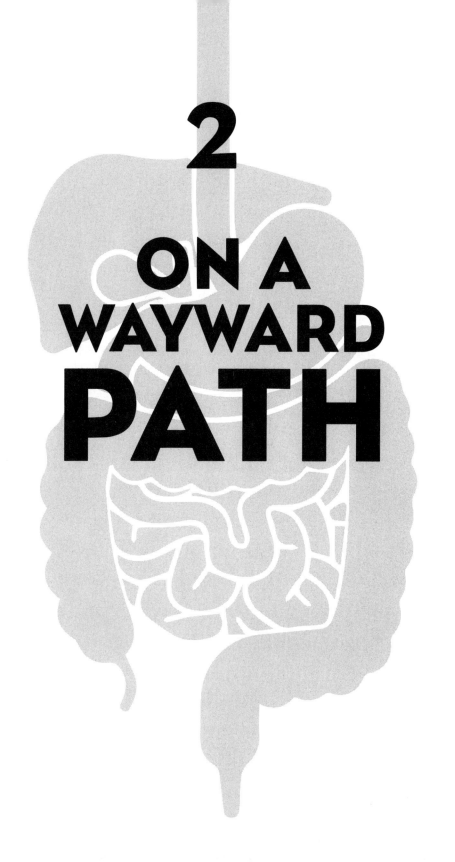

2

ON A WAYWARD PATH

HOW THE INTESTINE GETS SICK
AND SICKENS YOU

It's not only our eating behavior that makes our feces what they are. That would be too easy; reality is more complicated. Thorough chewing, no snacking, and a small dinner make a good foundation for proper digestion and healthy nourishment. If, however, we eat produce that is hard for the intestines to digest, they suffer. Oftentimes, it's not even a specific food we eat that causes trouble, but rather the amount we eat.

That Can Hurt! Milk, Bread, and Fruit— It Depends on the Amount

Many people have problems with lactose in dairy products such as milk, yogurt, cream, or ice cream. The lactase enzyme necessary to break down lactose is not produced after childhood in 80 percent of human beings. If we cannot break down lactose, the small intestine cannot absorb it. Which means it lands in the large intestine as bacteria food and ferments. Flatulence and diarrhea are the consequences.

Another nutritional component that causes trouble for many people is the gluten found in grain products, like bread or pasta. For 1 percent of people, gluten irritates their intestinal villi so badly that it triggers a violent immune reaction that can lead to diarrhea, among other things. The villi become partially destroyed and are no longer capable of absorbing essential nutrients. The reaction is not always this extreme.

We usually don't even notice that our bowels get increasingly tired after regular contact with gluten. Gluten is also able to undo the connections between the intestinal cells—cell junctions—causing the intestines to absorb nutrients that they shouldn't.

More and more people with worn-out intestines are having trouble digesting fructose, a sugar that appears in large quantities in fruit. It makes its way into the large intestine, where it ferments. This makes us pass gas tremendously, and fireworks go off in our stomach. The intestines don't feel like thickening anymore, so they send the fermenting pulp outside as quickly as possible. The fermentation and putrefaction processes cause a wild party for bacteria and uncontrolled production of toxins. This progressively weakens the bowel and makes room for intestinal tumors and vascular calcifications.

In this part, you will learn what consequences this process has on your bowel, intestinal flora, liver, skin, every single cell, your psyche, and even your spinal cord.

Milk Does a Body Good—Pass It On

A lot of you probably remember the slogan "Milk—it does a body good" from the eighties. Back then, like today, the milk industry had to come up with an ad campaign to reach potential customers. However, milk is only a staple in infants' or toddlers' diets. Adults barely need milk and other dairy products.

And please, milk does not do a body good. A man is tired, lying relaxed on the sofa in front of the TV, and drinks a glass of milk. After an hour at the latest, right when he is about to fall asleep, his intestines start to grumble and gurgle. Wanting to avoid any accidents, he runs to the toilet and frees himself of the fermenting irritant.

It's the lactase's fault, the enzyme 80 percent of the adult population no longer produces. We need this enzyme to decompose the lactose in milk. Lactose is a disaccharide sugar. A disaccharide is a double sugar made by condensation of one molecule of each of the simple sugars glucose and galactose. In order to digest these sugars, the enzyme must undo this condensation, because the intestines are not able to absorb double sugars.

For this reason, the lactose is passed on, undigested, to the large intestine, where it ends up as bacteria fodder. During metabolization, the bacteria produce hydrogen, carbon dioxide, and fatty acids. These irritate the intestine; hence, it wants to get rid of them as soon as possible. The carbon dioxide can lead to a stomachache and cramps if it causes excessive bloating in the intestinal loops. The extra hydrogen is absorbed by the intestine and exhaled through our lungs.

And this is how lactose intolerance is detected: In the morning, 50 grams (1.76 ounces) of lactose is administered on an empty stomach. Every thirty minutes after that, the person blows into a small device that measures the concentration of hydrogen in his or her breath. If the person is lactose intolerant, the concentration increases after about one to three hours.

In the United States, about 25 percent of the population is not able to digest dairy products, and 80 percent worldwide. Some people assume that the entire human race was lactose intolerant up until about 5000 BC. We weren't genetically predisposed to digest milk after toddlerhood, because it is really only meant to feed babies. Genetically regulated, the production of lactase stops after a few years of life.

As humans began to harness and sometimes milk herd animals, gene mutation occurred in parts of Europe. People were able to drink milk at an advanced age without getting diarrhea. These mutations were predominantly passed on and slowly spread in this way, but they haven't reached, for instance, the Mediterranean region yet.

That is why in a country like Greece, no one drank milk up until a few years ago. Dairy products, on the other hand, were eaten and tolerated as long as bacteria could break down the lactose in an adequately long maturation process.

Greek yogurt matures for a long time in a cup, thus making it tolerable. For the same reason, aged cheese contains little lactose and is therefore unproblematic for most lactose-intolerant people. Due to globalization of food products, fresh milk arrived in Greece and other Mediterranean countries, but often resulted in bloating and mushy stools for those who consumed it.

In Africa and Asia, someone who can tolerate milk is an exception to the rule. Almost 100 percent of the people there are lactose intolerant, meaning that after the age of four or five, they can no longer drink milk without experiencing diarrhea and bloating. Milk chocolate would be the wrong housewarming gift, and not only because of the hot weather.

Even if many people in the Western world are genetically able to drink milk, this ability decreases with age. The older and more worn-out an intestine is, the less lactase it produces. For years, you may have enjoyed and easily tolerated drinking cappuccino, and then suddenly you start getting gas and diarrhea.

In that case, the milk slogan should actually read, "Milk wears a body down—pass it on!"

In 2012, the milk industry was able to convince the Turkish government that its seven million children were not drinking enough milk, whatever "too little" according to the industry was. The government started the largest nutrition program in its history. Every child received at least one free milk box from day one. And on day one, thousands of children ended up in the hospital (some were even rushed over in ambulances) due to extreme nausea, stomachaches, and diarrhea. Turkey belongs to those countries where almost everyone is lactose intolerant. They could have seen the problems coming; nevertheless, the government decided to stick to this program. It's hard to imagine what arguments convinced them to do so.

Fermentation irritates the large intestine. The massive resulting gas production can render the valve that protects the small intestine from an invasion of bacteria inoperable. If the small intestine gets sick because bacteria spread in large amounts, the condition is called *bacterial overgrowth*. This means that fermentation has already started in the small intestine. The grumbling and gurgling starts fifteen minutes to half an hour after consuming milk, which damages the otherwise-busy intestinal villi, and our supply of nutrients and vitamins becomes worse and worse.

Lactose in dairy products is not the only problem. Casein, a milk protein, also carries certain risks. Some people are allergic to it as babies. This can lead to cradle cap, the first sign of a future full of allergies. How babies become allergic, no one knows for sure. We do know that some people have difficulties breaking down and digesting the casein in cow milk.

Homogenized milk can provoke yet another health problem. Homogenization breaks down fat molecules in milk from about 2 to 10 micrometers (μm) to about 0.2 to 0.5 μm by pressing the milk through a valve at high pressure. To give you an idea of these dimensions, the diameter of a hair is about 100 μm. The molecules are broken down to such a small size that they remain suspended evenly throughout the milk instead of rising to the top and creating a layer of cream.

Homogenization makes milk clearer and also more tolerable. In their original size, the larger fat molecules are hard for humans to digest. Enzymes called lipases work to break down the fat molecules, but they have a hard time with the larger ones.

The large, undigested fat molecules reach the large intestine by breaking down into free fatty acids and hydroxy fatty acids. These acids irritate the mucous membrane and lead to diarrhea. This is why milk was a problem before homogenization, even for those people who could produce lactase. Pretty much everyone got diarrhea. After homogenization, consumers were happy, and sales rose due to better tolerance. However, the same thing that boosted sales also hurt our health.

With the achievement of homogenization came a new problem: During animal testing, intestines reacted to this industrially modified milk with an immune response that released a lot of histamines. Histamines are essential for the defense against foreign substances in the body; too many can produce allergies. Some consequences of homogenization were skin allergies and asthma, and the intestine became enlarged.

The allergic reactions cannot be directly blamed on the small fat molecules. One hypothesis posits that many little fat molecules surround complex proteins, like a Trojan horse, and the proteins can escape digestion in the stomach this way. They sneak into the small intestine, where they provoke an immune response.

If we were to reduce our consumption of dairy products for the abovementioned reasons, our intestines would feel better, but what about our bones? After all, we were hounded into believing that milk delivers the calcium we need for our bones. We were told that we are the only living beings that needed milk from other living beings until a ripe old age; otherwise, we'd get osteoporosis and our bones would break.

Luckily, that isn't true! If milk could truly protect our bones from degenerating, there should be very few cases of osteoporosis in countries like America, Austria, Switzerland, Germany, and other countries in the Western world.

Yet when we take a closer look at these countries, we realize that the more dairy products consumed, the higher the osteoporosis rate. In a Swedish study carried out in 2014 on over sixty thousand women and forty-five thousand men (the men were observed for thirteen years and the women for over twenty-two years), it was shown that, especially in women, a higher dairy consumption correlated with more frequent bone fractures and even increased mortality rate. In conclusion, a balanced, diversified diet with mostly vegetables, legumes, and nuts contains enough calcium to keep our bones strong until old age. Weight-bearing physical activity and sunlight also keep our bones from breaking.

It will still take a while before we discover all the mechanisms that make milk one of the most significant allergens, but it's clear that an allergic reaction to casein in early childhood starts a lifelong battle with allergies. We also need more time to understand why women's bones become more porous due to milk and why they die earlier. In the meantime, there's no need to hide in the corner every time someone offers you a latte. And you don't need to do without a delicious old cheese if it's staring at you.

What's important is to pay attention in daily life to the quality of the dairy products. They should be unmodified if possible (that is to say, probably labeled "raw"), and you should try to forgo large daily quantities. If you get gassy after a latte, consider that it may be the result of lactose intolerance. And if you suddenly suffer from inexplicable eczema, it's a good idea to remember that milk protein could be the culprit.

Our Daily Bread

Of all things, it's our daily bread that makes our intestines squirm, or at least what humans have done to our bread in the past decades. Cereals didn't always accompany our meals. If we put the entire history of mankind on two hundred feet worth of letter-size sheets of paper, cereals would appear on the last sheet of our diet history.

For the most part, humans were happy eating what they hunted or gathered. They probably had already noticed that some birds lived off of grains. They must have discovered, after trying to imitate the birds, that their digestive tracts couldn't handle it. They could see the undigested kernels in their feces, which only helped spread the cereal.

Anything that comes out like it went in is not nourishment. Our ancestors must have wondered how they could break the grain down into really tiny pieces. They needed heat to make it digestible; that much they knew. That was a good ten thousand years ago, and still not everyone has managed to adapt to this relatively new food. For centuries, we ground it into flour and fed the components that were hard to digest to the pigs, until an organic fad in the 1970s taught us better. Fiber in fruit and vegetables became popular, but they were also placed on the same level with whole-grain products.

We should've known that something wasn't right when our gas production cranked up. Many people thought the flatulence was a sign of a new, healthy lifestyle and, therefore, considered it something positive. But the label "hard to digest" that many whole-grain products carry is not the only reason that grains make some intestines' lives difficult.

The blame also lies with gluten, a mix of proteins that is found in most kinds of grains. Its name comes from Latin and means "glue." If we knead dough and then add a lot of water, it ends up like one huge piece of gum, which is the gluten. The gas that comes from baking the added yeast blows up the many little pieces of chewing gum (gluten) that are spread throughout the dough. This is how fluffy bread is created.

In recent years, the gluten in wheat—the most commonly used grain—has tripled due to special breeding techniques used to produce grain that will make the bread fluffier. The consumer loves it this way, so the industry makes it possible. Fresh low-gluten bread often has the same consistency as old gluten-rich bread. The low-gluten bread becomes harder and tougher to chew, which many consumers find unappealing. And mechanically produced dough is easier to manufacture when it contains as much gluten as possible (as many bubble-building pieces of chewing gum as possible).

Another reason our tolerance might be suffering is because humans have extensively changed wheat in just a few years, something nature could never have achieved in thousands of years. Of course, change in general is not bad. What would life be like without change? It depends on which changes we accept and which ones we should try to avoid.

It's not always just gluten in wheat products that makes our intestines struggle. Professor Detlef Schuppan at the University of Mainz searched for a year to find additional possible culprits, and he did. The wheat industry had bred a protein by the name of *adenosine triphosphate amylase* into the modern super-wheat to defend against vermin, but it may also cause problems for our intestines. Somehow, no one suspected that something that works so well as an insecticide and helps increase sales could also harm our intestines.

Consequently, we should avoid this modern, modified wheat if we want to care for our intestines and health in general. You can find wheat in organic grocery stores that hasn't been exposed to these changes.

Celiac disease

If you have celiac disease, your small intestine makes the decision on whether gluten is good or bad. In the United States, one in every 133 people has this life-changing illness, and just twenty-five years ago, it was one in a thousand. You can tell this disease is on the rise by looking at the gluten-free section in your local supermarket. The more wheat that is consumed in a country, the more cases of celiac disease can be found.

In Turkey, almost 441 pounds of bread is consumed per person each year, resulting in the highest occurrence of celiac disease—1.5 out of

100 people. Germany and Ireland tie for consumption of bread at 176 pounds per person. Most would have guessed that the French eat the largest amount of bread, probably because we see them with baguettes under their arms in our French-language books, and no other nation is linked to a type of bread as much as France. But the French's bread consumption lies more in the middle, at 132 pounds per person. Americans, on average, consume 53 pounds of bread per person, per year.

Why are these proteins—gluten—so damaging for some intestines?

If someone with celiac desease tries food containing gluten for the first time, in a little while, it will trigger a pronounced immune response in the bowel as it tries to fight against the protein in gluten called gliadin. The reaction is so bad that the intestinal villi in the small intestine eventually become severely damaged and, after years of no treatment, are completely destroyed. This can lead to fatty stool, because the consumed fat in food can no longer be digested. Diarrhea and vomiting may occur, and the body slowly degenerates, because iron, folic acid, zinc, and vitamins A, E, K, D, and B12 can no longer be properly absorbed.

In a healthy bowel, the intestinal mucous membrane controls what the body absorbs and what must remain in the intestine. A damaged intestinal mucosa becomes permeable to gliadin, so patients with celiac disease have a higher quantity of gliadin bodies in their blood. How this affects the course of the disease is not yet known.

What we do know is that the immune system produces antibodies against intestinal muscle proteins (transglutaminase and endomysium) in about 90 percent of celiac disease patients. So not only does the immune response to gluten damage the intestines, but it also damages the immune system itself, as it directly attacks the bowel. Many other autoimmune diseases (when the immune system attacks its own body's tissues) are more frequently found in patients with celiac disease. Examples of these diseases are type 1 diabetes, rheumatoid arthritis, and Hashimoto's thyroiditis. Diseases where the intestine is chronically inflamed, such as ulcerative colitis and Crohn's disease, are also more common, but even asthma and eczema have been linked to celiac disease. You can compare it to a watchdog that was trained to viciously attack invaders, but now attacks anyone with two legs, even his owner (who represents our organs).

Improved diagnostics surely has something to do with the increase in celiac disease patients. They've also helped us to realize that not every person with the disease suffers from diarrhea. Most adult patients consult their doctors for extreme fatigue, nerve pain, bleeding tendency, or edema (swelling) before knowing what they have. Therefore, it's a good idea to consider celiac disease when these symptoms occur and to test for the corresponding antibodies in your blood.

Unfortunately, it's not just bread, gluten, and adenosine triphosphate amylase that make our intestinal mucosa work overtime.

Open Sesame

Immunological reactions and intestinal mucosal damage are not the only things that make the intestines permeable to foreign proteins.

About ten years ago, a protein was discovered that the bowel itself creates and that modulates the permeability of tight junctions between cells of the wall of the digestive tract. Its name is *zonulin*. Due to this protein, all kinds of large molecules can enter the intestine. These large molecules should not leave the intestines and enter the blood; otherwise, the immune system will identify them as foreign and start to defend us against them.

Again, in blood tests of patients with autoimmune diseases like type 1 diabetes, rheumatoid arthritis, Hashimoto's thyroiditis, and chronic inflammatory intestinal diseases, such as ulcerative colitis and Crohn's disease, the level of zonulin in the blood and stool rises. Zonulin is a kind of "open sesame" for all kinds of foreign invaders that shouldn't be in our blood and may cause us harm.

The question remains why the damaged intestine creates a protein whose impact wreaks havoc on the entire organism. We're going to have to wait a while for that answer. Luckily, we are now able to determine the level of zonulin in our blood through a simple blood or stool test, allowing us to see if and how badly our intestines are damaged.

WHEN APPLES CAUSE FLATULENCE

In the cases of milk and wheat, we are dealing with foods that may cause harm to the intestines. They haven't been on the human menu for very long, and if we were to reduce their intake tomorrow, no one would care, and our intestines may even smile again.

But what about fruits? Over the history of mankind, they've always been on our menu and praised for all their vitamins. Yet can it be they may cause problems as well?

Yes! Because problems may occur if the fructose in the fruit cannot be digested well. There is an extremely rare type of fructose intolerance where the body is able to absorb the fructose yet cannot break it down normally due to a congenital enzyme defect. This leads to liver and kidney damage as well as hypoglycemia.

If a patient is diagnosed with *fructose malabsorption* (sometimes falsely labeled *fructose intolerance*), it's a whole other story. In this case, the absorption of fructose in the intestines is disrupted. The cause lies in a poorly developed or overworked transport system.

This merits a closer look: Fructose is a simple sugar, which is carried by one of the many specialized transport system channels from the intestines into or through the cells. The first transport system ever discovered carries glucose (also a simple sugar) into the blood cells and was therefore called GLUT1. So far, fourteen more of these transport systems have been found. The one responsible for transporting fructose through the intestinal cells is called GLUT5, because it was the fifth one to be discovered. Healthy intestines with a functioning transport system are able to transfer 30 to 40 grams (1 to 1.5 ounces) of fructose daily. If even more fructose ends up in the small intestine, it cannot be transported, in other words absorbed, and is sent straight to the large intestine, where it finishes as bacteria fodder. You can compare the transport system with a bus, which has a finite number of seats. When the buses are full, the rest of the passengers have to remain outside.

The bacteria are delighted to receive the extra portion of sugar, which ferments into alcohol, carbon dioxide, hydrogen, and fatty acids, which explains the typical complaints from those who experience fructose malabsorption. Carbon dioxide causes flatulence, the fatty acids often cause diarrhea, and the hydrogen is used for diagnostics. Like the test for lactose intolerance, it appears almost instantly in the exhaled air and can be detected if the patient blows into a small device.

Up until a few decades ago, fructose malabsorption was never a problem, because we didn't eat a lot of fructose. For a long time, the average daily consumption of fructose was 15 grams (0.53 ounces). An apple contains about 10 to 15 grams (0.35 to 0.53 ounces) of fructose. Fruit was seasonal, and if you did eat too much of it and got gassy, you just ate less the next time.

These days, doctors recommend eating fruit or vegetables at least five times per day. If you choose fruit over vegetables, your transport system is quickly overwhelmed with work, and you feel discomfort even though you thought you were doing everything right. Furthermore, we eat oodles of fructose without even realizing it. For instance, when "no added sugar" is written on a jar of jam, it still contains fructose. And the list goes on and on when it comes to industrially manufactured foods.

An interesting question is why the transport of fructose is limited at all. Fructose, like alcohol, is metabolized in the liver and, again like alcohol, can be toxic in large quantities. Among other problems, it can lead to fatty liver disease (FLD). Therefore, limiting our consumption is a wise idea.

But how is it possible that people get nonalcoholic fatty liver disease if only a limited amount of fructose can be absorbed? White granulated sugar is a double sugar (disaccharide), consisting of two simple sugars, fructose and glucose. Glucose nourishes all our cells. The intestines absorb it with barely any limitations. White granulated sugar is broken down in the intestines into its two simple sugars, and the fructose sneaks onto the bus that was supposed to be carrying only glucose. This is how fructose can find its way to the liver as a hidden passenger.

Sorbitol, an industry-favored sugar substitute, blocks the transportation of fructose entirely. It would be as if the bus were on a test run, so no one was allowed to get on. This means that fructose is no longer absorbed at all, and the discomfort is accordingly intensified.

Until now, we've only talked about too many people wanting to get on the bus without a seat. However, there are some intestinal diseases or afflictions that force the body to only use small buses, so the capacity is reduced. Gluten intolerance is an example of this kind of intestinal affliction, as well as the presence of incompatible bacteria in the small intestines. How is this all related?

Let's imagine that gluten weakens the bowel and, therefore, fewer and smaller buses are running and the fructose cannot be absorbed entirely. This leads to strong fermentation processes in the ascending colon. The resulting gases hurt the valve between the small and large intestines. It can no longer entirely close. Germs from the large intestine can now settle more and more in the small intestine, which increasingly loses strength and health.

Research from various countries reveals that a third of humans exhibit incomplete absorption of fructose after eating 25 grams (0.88 ounces). This means that the 30 to 40 grams that are considered normal are way too much for many people.

Only half of fructose-intolerant people display the typical discomforts (flatulence and diarrhea) which are, more often than not, the cause of irritable bowel syndrome. The other half have bacteria that aren't that excited about fructose and, therefore, induce less fermentation. Now, you're probably thinking that the latter half got lucky. Unfortunately, that's not the case, because fructose malabsorption comes with a few other issues.

Flatulence and diarrhea are only symptoms of a tired or sick bowel that is no longer capable of absorbing fructose. And as we've observed, sick intestines fail at absorbing not only fructose, but also other nutrients and vitamins.

More and more people with fructose intolerance and malabsorption are suffering from depression. It's believed their intestines also struggle with absorbing tryptophan, since tryptophan is found in smaller quantities than usual in the blood of fructose-intolerant people. Tryptophan is converted in the brain to serotonin, which is known as the "happy hormone." Less tryptophan in the blood means less serotonin in the brain, and our mood sinks.

We've all heard before that a little chocolate enhances our mood. When we eat something sweet, the pancreas produces insulin to metabolize the sugar. It has been proven that insulin can do even more. For instance, it improves the absorption of tryptophan in the brain. This is clearly not the solution for depression that is caused by worn-out intestines, especially because of the eventual weight gain. But you can see the connection now.

A lack of folic acid and zinc are other signs of fructose malabsorption. If these deficiencies—as well as depression—appear, it makes sense to drastically reduce your fructose consumption, at least for a while. My fitness program for your intestines improves the absorption of tryptophan, folic acid, and zinc, and life is grand once again.

Now you understand why dairy products, bread, and fruit are to be enjoyed with caution. Yet there's no reason to panic and quit eating it all. It's the amount of these foods we consume that matters. *Everything in moderation* is a good idea.

Histamines

There is another substance that can cause mayhem in our bodies if our intestines are worn out—histamine. As previously mentioned, this substance is produced by our own bodies; it is found in living creatures and plants, and even bacteria can create it. It's a jack-of-all-trades, which can be good and bad, as you'll soon see.

The list of possible symptoms is long—headache, migraine, a stuffed-up or runny nose, rapid and irregular heartbeat, premature ventricular contraction (PVC), soft stool to diarrhea, low blood pressure, swollen eyes, red blotches on the body or face, and urticaria (hives). These can all be signs that your body can no longer tolerate certain foods. The trigger in this case is the histamine, which is found in large quantities in ripe produce and created by bacterial processes.

Histamines are significant for the body's defense against foreign substances and are also the most significant inflammatory substances for pathological allergic diseases and asthma. Histamines enlarge the blood vessels and make the uterus contract. They are what trigger contractions during pregnancy.

Let's delve into that last sentence a little further. The placenta produces an enzyme to prevent contractions. This enzyme, amine oxidase, is able to break down histamines. Pregnant women have about five hundred times more of this enzyme in their blood than nonpregnant women.

A healthy small intestine can also produce enough of this enzyme to neutralize histamines in food or those made by bacteria in the colon. Otherwise, the abovementioned symptoms could arise.

Sick intestines cannot produce enough enzymes, and alcohol and some medications reduce the quantity of enzymes created as well. If histamines reach the intestinal mucosa, amine oxidase is there to save the day. And if this isn't enough, the liver initiates one last attempt to put out the fire by creating an enzyme called N-methyltransferase. You could compare this enzyme with firefighters who are on the lookout for fire hazards to prevent disasters.

How can we apply this concept to daily life? Let's assume that your intestines are working well, and the amine oxidase production in the intestinal cells is sufficient. One evening, you eat some histamine-rich food, like a tuna steak, some aged cheese, and one or more glasses of red wine to wash it all down. Firstly, the red wine is full of histamines, and secondly, the alcohol disarms the firefighters in your intestines. We often feel the effects of red wine as a stuffy nose or a headache the next day. A low-histamine white wine, on the other hand, might have saved you from feeling those effects.

If you've ever experienced diarrhea or circulatory problems after eating spoiled food, it might have been due to the large quantities of histamines. The next day, you usually feel much better. However, if it goes on for days, you should question the bacteria contained in the spoiled food.

If you only show signs of one of the abovementioned symptoms, you may be about to discover if the food is overly ripe or your intestines are worn out and no longer able to provide enough firefighters. It's also conceivable that alcohol or medication reduced the number of fire department units. Or you ate certain foods we call *histamine liberators* that trigger allergies, which is why your body released histamines.

There's an easy way to find out. For one week, don't eat any foods that are high in histamines, and do without alcohol and foods you're allergic to. Before you start, have your doctor test for the levels of histamine and amine oxidase in your blood. The results are not always clear, so take into account the weeklong break.

Regarding histamines in my intestinal fitness program, I've listed valuable information that will help you maintain a balanced bowel flora.

Histamine-containing foods
- aged cheese +++
- salami and other cold cuts +++
- fish if it's not freshly caught +++
- red wine vinegar +++
- sauerkraut +++
- tomatoes +
- spinach +

Histamine-containing alcoholic drinks
- red wine +++
- champagne +++
- wheat beer ++
- white wine +
- beer +

Amine oxidase inhibitors (a full list can be found online)
- alcohol
- acetylcysteine (loosens thick mucus)
- ambroxol

- aminophylline
- amitriptyline
- chloroquine
- clavulanic acid
- isoniazid
- metamizole
- metoclopramide
- propafenone
- verapamil

Histamine liberators (substances in food that trigger the production of histamines)
- chocolate
- potentially citrus fruits, strawberries, kiwis, nuts

FLORA AND FAUNA—AS LONG AS THE BACTERIA ARE HARMLESS

What we eat is not the only thing that can damage our intestines. Which microorganisms grow in our bowels and what this growth releases can affect our intestines and, as a result, our health.

Lately, it seems like everyone is talking about intestinal flora. What is that all about?

The intestinal flora is the entirety of all microorganisms in the intestines. Those who have decided to improve their health and intestinal flora try eating probiotic yogurt (a yogurt full of living microorganisms), kimchi, and so on.

Flora was the Roman goddess of spring, flowers, and youth. In Latin, flora means "flower." In modern scientific terms, it means "plant life." So the question arises: What is it doing in our bowels? Not such a long time ago, bacteria were considered plants, and the term *intestinal flora* harkens to those times. Amoeba and worms, which can easily get lost in our intestines, technically belong in the category of intestinal fauna (the animal world). But that would just make everything more complicated. Therefore, everyone sticks with the term intestinal flora, which denotes the entirety of bacteria, fungi, parasites, viruses, and more that live in our intestines.

Approximately one thousand types of bacteria can multiply in our intestines. In fact, every single one of us has a mixed bouquet of about three hundred exquisite kinds. We don't know what about half of them look like, because we cannot get them to grow outside the intestine. And why our bodies specifically chose these three hundred, we don't know either. We assume that it has something to do with what germs we came into contact with from birth on. Babies born by cesarean have different germs than children born vaginally, who came into contact with germs in the birth canal.

Overall, each of us carries about one hundred trillion bacteria in our intestines; that's 100,000,000,000,000! If your intestinal bacteria were tulips, and you planted one of your tulips per square foot, then you could cover the entire United States in tulips.

Do you feel like a little bacteria history? About two hundred years ago, soon after European scientists discovered intestinal bacteria, they tried to find out if these bacteria were good for us, had no influence on us at all, or could potentially cause damage.

Louis Pasteur, a French chemist and microbiologist, performed research in 1880 on animals that were fed only sterilized food to see if they could survive without intestinal bacteria. Guess what. They couldn't! He concluded that the intestinal flora was vital for humans. At the same time, he was well aware of how dangerous bacteria could be outside our intestines. Unfortunately, however, he had no clue that vitamins existed. Therefore, he failed to realize that he took away the animals' chance of survival by sterilizing the food and destroying the vitamins. And because surgery was still at an early stage, he couldn't have known that a person who has lost his or her colon, along with all its living germs, due to sickness or serious accident can still lead a long, healthy life.

At the beginning of the twentieth century, after vitamins were proven essential, some claimed that bacteria were necessary for providing us with vitamins.

By the time it was proven in the 1930s that intestinal flora is not at all necessary, that intestinal germs consume more vitamins than they produce, and that strong toxins are produced when they break down indigestible or poorly digested food pulp, it was already too late. It couldn't change people's minds about what scientists had been saying for decades—and it was clear that it would take decades to eradicate these beliefs.

For the last ten years, exhaustive research has been conducted about the influence of the intestinal flora on our bodies. Intestinal bacteria are not necessary but practically inevitable. Therefore, we have to learn to live with them.

What's important is that they don't cause any harm. In other words, they need to be harmless. But what does a harmless intestinal flora look like?

We know that we have flora—bacteria—in our mouths, but our stomachs are almost germ-free because of the strong acidic environment where germs don't feel comfortable. We know that barely any germs make it out alive from a healthy stomach because it is an acidic hell for them.

If, however, the stomach is sick or receives very poorly chewed food, the germs have a chance of making it into the small intestine. Over time, we'll be continuously confronted with new germs that can settle in our intestines if the environment is right and our defenses are down. Among those germs that make it, there is a good chance that a few of them are evildoers.

A healthy small intestine is practically germ-free as well—at least, the first half of it is. But when the valve between the small and large intestine cannot close entirely, germs from the large intestine can creep in. It's still nothing to worry about, since the small intestine has natural defenses against bacterial growth.

When it is weak, however, it loses this defense capability, and we get sick. As you already know, this disorder is called *bacterial overgrowth*. The bacteria tackle the food pulp in the small intestine before it can be well digested and its nutrients sent to the body in the blood. This can lead to malnutrition, deficiencies, painful joints, and much more.

Normally, the germs tackle leftovers in their ancestral home first—the large intestine. These digestive leftovers dictate which germs and how many of them exist, which then determines if the intestinal flora is harmless or harmful. The following is an example of intestinal flora.

Infants that were fed mother's milk have an entirely different intestinal flora than babies that were fed cow milk. The difference between mother's milk and cow milk proteins alone (the latter being a little harder to digest) attracts bacteria—which love to metabolize—to what we haven't digested. Bottle-fed babies often have more trouble with their intestines, their stool begins to stink, and they have more allergies later in life.

There's also new research that shows that rotting, poorly digested chicken eggs produce toxins that cause arteriosclerosis (arterial calcification). Another troubling strain on our intestinal flora is when we send poorly chewed meat or large amounts of it into the large intestine. The putrefaction bacteria in our colon feel especially comfortable, so they produce . . . cancer-causing putrefaction toxins! The risk of colon cancer rises. Yet the simultaneous intake of fiber-rich foods can lower the risk of cancer once more, because the fibers partially absorb the putrefaction toxins and speed up the intestinal passage time, which minimizes reactions on the intestinal wall. That just goes to show us how complex everything is in the large intestine!

Due to bad eating habits, some people have managed to create intestinal flora that is world champion in converting everything—literally everything—into calories. And then they get fat. You're surely familiar with the alarming rise in overweight people in developed countries. The intestinal flora may contribute to weight gain, but for the most part, the amount we eat and how we eat remain the decisive factors.

We might be able to manipulate the intestinal flora a little by eating intestinal germs, against all better judgment. However, a better way to improve it is by changing our diet. We should change how we eat and, eventually, what we eat as well.

The idea of growing bacteria in our colons by eating harmless intestinal germs in yogurt or other probiotic foods and medications has been around for a long time. *Probiotic* means living microorganisms, like the lactic acid bacteria in yogurt or microbes in yeast, sauerkraut, and other items. These attempts are often useless because the germs can't make it through a healthy stomach. The acids kill them off. They would have to be able to neutralize, at least temporarily, the acids with alkaline substances. Besides, the bacteria need a special environment, suitable for their growth.

In 1892, Max von Pettenkofer, a Bavarian hygienist, pursued this idea by swallowing one cubic centimeter of a fresh culture of pure cholera bacteria in order to prove that the environment plays a decisive role in bacterial growth. Shortly beforehand, he drank a glass of water mixed with baking soda, an alkaline powder, to cancel out the acidic environment in his stomach and allow for the cholera bacteria to enter his intestines. He didn't get sick. It's amazing what people will do when they're convinced of something.

It's just as difficult to colonize cholera bacteria in a healthy bowel as it is to make sure that harmless bacteria feel well and reproduce in a sick intestine.

When we have healthy intestines and carry around masses of harmless intestinal germs, harmful germs have a hard time settling in because they don't love a healthy environment. A harmless intestinal flora is almost like an extra immune system. The germs are not at all interested in sharing their fodder, not to mention their usual spot, with evil invaders.

As soon as we start to crank up fermentation and putrefaction processes through bad dietary habits and eating endless amounts of food, the environment in our intestines changes, and it gets easier and easier for pests to multiply.

You can determine which kind of bacteria are allowed to thrive and which ones aren't by changing how, when, and what you eat. A fitness program for your intestines tries to thin out your intestinal flora, reduce fermentation and putrefaction, and, in the end, change the intestinal environment. There's more information about that in part 3.

The Antibiotic Dilemma

What and how we eat determines significantly whether we carry a harmless intestinal flora around with us or one that harms us. Natural enemies of this flora are malignant, disease-causing germs that can outsmart all defense mechanisms. We usually end up with diarrheal diseases as a result. If the germs manage to push their way into our bodies, they can lead to serious, life-threatening diseases.

But that's not all. There is a group of medications that create trouble for our intestines. They are called *antibiotics*. They are a blessing for the human race but, oftentimes, a disaster for our intestinal friends.

Before the Scottish bacteriologist Alexander Fleming went on vacation in the summer of 1928, he injected an agar plate with bacteria. Agar plates are Petri dishes that contain a growth medium (typically agar plus nutrients) used to culture microorganisms. When he returned, he discovered that besides bacteria, mold had grown in the plate, and everywhere in the vicinity of the mold, bacteria had not multiplied. That specific mold in Latin was called *Penicillium notatum*, which led Fleming to call his new bacteria-killing substance *penicillin*. He learned that this toxin killed certain bacteria but wasn't poisonous for human or animal cells. The idea of fighting disease with this discovery didn't enter his mind.

Almost ten years went by before an Australian, Howard Florey, and a German, Ernst Boris Chain, both working in England, stumbled upon Fleming's discovery while searching for antibiotic substances. In 1940, penicillin was tested on a human for the first time as a treatment against a lethal infection.

Despite Florey and Chain's efforts, the amount of penicillin wasn't enough for a successful treatment. After the penicillin lowered the fever for a short period, the patient's health worsened again, and he eventually died of the infection. Still, demand for the drug rose—but is was difficult to produce. There was so little available at the time that they extracted it from the urine of treated patients for resuse. Shortly thereafter, industrial production of penicillin began. Since the end of the Second World War, during which large quantities were needed for war injuries, there have been enough antibiotics in Europe for everyone.

After the 1940s, researchers developed more antibiotics against germs that were resistant to penicillin, saving many people's lives. Soon, we were capable of treating almost every bacterial disease successfully.

Two examples of diseases that were usually lethal before the invention of antibiotics are puerperal fever and heart valve disease. Or an infected hangnail could have easily lead to the amputation of the whole leg. And success in surgery depended on antibiotics to prevent the wounds from getting infected.

There was another side to the coin, though: because antibiotics were so effective, doctors started using them for infections that weren't complicated or life-threatening. Simple influenza infections, which are caused by viruses (antibiotics are useless against viruses!), were being treated, along with uncomplicated bronchial infections, ear infections, bladder infections, and much more.

Furthermore, large quantities of antibiotics were being added to animal feed, which we then consumed in our meat. That's the way bacteria learned to bypass these new toxins. Many became resistant to previously lethal substances. They're really good at that.

Bacteria have colonized our earth for about three billion years now and have learned how to deal with adverse conditions. They are truly skilled survivors. If they're not resistant to the effects of some antibiotics from the beginning, they'll become resistant by randomly mutating. They are capable of defending themselves against toxins because of changes in their genetic material.

Imagine the following scenario: You apply an antibiotic to a Petri dish the size of your hand that contains ten billion bacteria—more bacteria than people on earth. All of them die except one, which is resistant to the antibiotic.

The next day, the dish is colonized with the offspring of the one bacteria that survived. One more day later, there are as many as there were before. It would take human beings about four hundred thousand years to do the same. It's survival of the fittest—humans and bacteria behave in the same way, though bacteria are a lot faster!

In recent years, increasingly more bacterial infections have been appearing that are resistant to the existing antibiotics. In a mere seventy years, bacteria have learned to bypass the toxins. The strongest have survived and passed down their attributes to their offspring.

A large portion of our intestinal germs have gotten accustomed to antibiotics. Toddlers' intestinal flora are already resistant to most antibiotics these days. The human intestinal flora has changed drastically in the last seventy years. Germs that we lived with in peace for a very long time were replaced with other antibiotic-resistant compadres. These changes are considered responsible for many allergies.

Diarrhea after taking antibiotics could be due to a damaged intestinal flora or the direct effect of some antibiotics on the intestinal wall (it becomes inflamed). When we're dealing with a life-threatening, complicated disease, we are all willing to accept these side effects. If we're dealing, however, with influenza or an uncomplicated bacterial infection, we should think long and hard before taking antibiotics!

THE TOXIC KITCHEN IN YOUR BOWEL— AFFECTING EVERYTHING FROM YOUR HEAD DOWN TO YOUR TOES

"All things are poison and nothing is without poison; the [dose] alone makes a thing poison," wrote the Swiss German doctor Philippus Aureolus Theophrastus Bombast von Hohenheim in 1538. He is known as Paracelsus in medical history. He was convinced that the intake of toxins is one of the five main causes of disease.

Toxins in our intestines emerge especially from microbial breakdown of poorly digested food. As a result of fermentation and putrefaction processes, propionic acid, acetic acid, butyric acid, ethanol, and amines are produced, as well as unpleasant-smelling, toxic gases such as ammonia and hydrogen sulfide. Let's delve into that witch's cauldron a little further, because it gets even worse!

Undigested remains are not the only victims of a microbial break-down. If the bowel is worn out and cannot absorb all the tryptophan, the substance rots, thereby producing a putrefaction toxin named *indole*. Indole and *skatole*, another putrefaction toxin, give our stools the stench we've all smelled before.

After the intestines absorb indole, it's passed on to the liver, where it's converted into indican, which we can detect in our blood and urine. Many years ago, the level of indican was measured when an intestinal obstruction was suspected. An intestinal obstruction triggers a rapid, massive putrefaction process, which a high level of indican in the blood can confirm.

The rapid increase of indican in the blood and urine due to intestinal obstruction can be ascribed to putrefaction caused by a backlog in the small intestine. The small intestine is designed for absorption. It absorbs twenty times more liquid a day than the large intestine. Unfortunately, it's very efficient at absorbing any existing putrefaction toxins as well. But even if we don't have intestinal obstructions, the indican level lets us know how much tryptophan has already decayed in the intestines and can no longer provide us with the "happy" hormone, serotonin.

Now you know how toxins arise in our intestines, but how does this affect our digestion and overall health?

Luckily, neither our intestines nor our bodies are completely defenseless when toxins attack. The defense begins in the intestines. During healthy digestion, very few toxins are produced in the large intestine. The intestinal mucosa is the first barrier that has to resist a toxic substance. If people with bad digestion and stinky feces don't suffer from complications, it's usually thanks to an intact defense response against these toxins in the large intestine.

It's another story if the valve between the small and large intestines is not functioning properly and toxin-producing bacterial processes move into the small intestine. As you already know, the small intestine is all about absorbing and not defending against bacterial toxins, which shouldn't even be there in the first place.

How can the intestines defend themselves? We can imagine it like this: The toxin irritates the intestinal mucous membrane, which over-reacts. The more toxins there are, the more violent the reaction. The mucous membrane produces a lot of secretion to wash away the toxin and to attack the toxin-producing bacteria.

At the same time, stronger-than-normal intestinal movements begin to transport the nasty stuff farther. We start hearing noises from our intestines like gurgling and burbling. Our stomach hurts. If the irritation is really severe, we get diarrhea. The goal is to eliminate the toxin as quickly as possible.

We're familiar with this from our childhood. We had to stay in bed with a warm water bottle on our tummies, and saltines and ginger ale supposedly calmed our intestines. Even today, for most of us, the memory of pain associated with saltines doesn't exactly make them our favorite snack, even if they did bring relief.

Unfortunately, no one told us we could've avoided an irritated bowel, along with the saltine crackers, if our eating behavior had been okay. No one explained, so we experienced a few more episodes of the same, which wore out our intestines.

How do our intestines get tired? It's simple: they no longer defend themselves, and the affected section of the intestines goes into a stage of subnormal function. They no longer create enough secretion. Your stomach no longer hurts. The tired intestinal mucosa no longer absorbs the nutrients entirely, which cranks up the production of new toxins while the undigested chyme is broken down by bacteria. Even the protective intestinal movements decrease. The sick mucous membrane that lost a part of its barrier function starts absorbing more and more toxins and sends them to the liver via the blood.

The liver is an important workstation, because it's our waste treatment plant. The liver has a lot to do, and we count on it to handle these new demands. Unfortunately, it doesn't always work like this. No street cleaner is happy about waking up every morning to a huge layer of garbage on the streets he left clean the night before. The street cleaner, like the liver, has his limits and gets tired, which slows down his performance. And like the street cleaner, the liver's performance slows down. More and more toxins manage to make it through the treatment plant and hurt our bodies.

What Am I, Chopped Liver?

Has your liver ever run across a cheap bottle of wine? At least you knew why you felt like crap the next day.

The liver is not only an important organ for detoxifying alcohol; all the toxins we ingest while eating or which we produce in our colons are on their way to our livers in our blood—that is, if they made it through the defense mechanism of the intestinal mucous membrane.

The liver attempts to make the toxins harmless for us. Often, there are several steps necessary. The final products of the detoxification are frequently more poisonous than the toxins themselves. The pharmaceutical industry uses this fact for some medications that are activated by this transformation in the liver.

What happens with alcohol in the liver is comparatively simple. First, it's converted into acetaldehyde by an enzyme called *alcohol dehydrogenase*. Acetaldehyde is a more poisonous cell toxin than alcohol. Another enzyme called *acetaldehyde dehydrogenase* breaks the acetaldehyde down into acetic acid, and this is broken down in the last step, called the *citric acid cycle*, into water and carbon dioxide, which are then eliminated.

If this transformation worked 100 percent, we wouldn't have a hangover after a night on the town, because we get it from the acetaldehyde. We also wouldn't get a fatty liver from consuming a lot of alcohol. Acetaldehyde inhibits the breakdown of fatty acids in the liver, yet promotes the production of fatty acids. In this context, even cirrhosis wouldn't exist, a slowly progressing disease in which healthy liver tissue is replaced with scar tissue. If everything worked perfectly, we wouldn't even have alcohol in our blood after a good glass of wine or beer. The alcohol wouldn't reach our brains, and no one would ever be tipsy. If we think about it, no one would probably even drink alcohol anymore.

In reality, things look a lot different. About 10 percent of the alcohol we drink manages to bypass the immediate conversion process. We call that taking advantage of the weak. Fusel alcohols (alcohols that contain more than two carbons) and other toxins that are created by the fermentation and putrefaction processes in our bowels are also taken care of in this way. Small amounts are neutralized without a problem; however, large amounts become problematic. Furthermore, not every person is the same when it comes to breaking down alcohol and other toxins in the liver.

In many Asian people, only a small amount (which is genetically determined) of the enzyme alcohol dehydrogenase is produced. If there are not sufficient amounts of one of the enzymes necessary for the breakdown of alcohol, that one glass of wine isn't fun anymore.

Getting back to the liver, in the Middle Ages, we thought that feelings and temperament came from the liver. Even back then, people felt like chopped liver at times. But what if we feel like chopped liver without having consumed a bottle of wine? We're not sure. Are we just in a bad mood? It could be because of liver poisoning originating in the intestines. In a sick bowel, toxins can be produced in quantities so large that the liver cells perish and cirrhosis of the liver emerges, without us even drinking one sip of alcohol.

Maybe the liver is just plain tired. What are typical signs of a tired liver? Fatigue, memory loss, difficulty concentrating, and reduced performance are all symptoms. Not counting when you drink alcohol, how many days a year do you feel like this even a little?

The liver loves regenerating more than any other organ we have. If a part dies off or is damaged somehow, new tissue is created. That sounds like a solid foundation. But even this organ can tire and get sick from overexertion.

There is still a lot of research to be done in order to show which intestinal toxins are completely broken down, by what, and how. And who is better or less capable, due to which genetic mutations, to neutralize this or that toxin? How do these bacterial toxins affect our bodies when they escape the detoxification program of the liver?

Are they the sole cause of certain diseases? These are questions that researchers have been asking for many years.

Hazardous Materials or Toxins?

Every year, right after the New Year, magazines and health websites write targeted articles for those who are determined to do something good for their health, and detoxing has been a hot topic for decades. We mainly see new detoxing methods reported positively in American media, but overseas we see plenty of headlines debunking or against detoxing, cleanses, or decontamination, as it's widely referred to in Europe. Headlines reading, "There's no such thing as a decontamination cleanse, because there is no such thing as contaminated people outside of hazardous zones. Therefore, cleansing is nonsense!" are pretty common and give the majority of the readers who didn't plan on doing anything for their health anyway feel vindicated.

And surprisingly these magazines would be right! There really is no such thing as natural decontamination in humans. But let's first define terms as clearly as possible to avoid confusion.

What exactly is decontamination? Human decontamination is the process of cleansing the human body to remove or neutralize contamination by hazardous materials, such as chemicals, radioactive substances, and infectious material.

If we stretched it a little, we could consider our feces contaminated. Hazardous material could describe many people's toilet experiences. However, the thought of something being radioactive inside us just doesn't serve as a good comparison. Our stool is not what "decontamination" programs are targeting, though.

Detoxification is the right word! Because obviously there are toxins in our bodies that our detoxification organs eliminate, through our kidneys, skin, liver, and intestines. We either eat these toxins or produce them through metabolic processes. Our sick bowels can also create them. They only partially absorb these toxins and, unfortunately, don't always eliminate them immediately.

Even if we don't carry hazardous material around in our bodies, toxins definitely develop in the intestines. Some are a result of metabolizing vital substances. The sicker our intestines, the more of these poisonous substances are produced and absorbed. Thse toxins have proven effects on our intestines, liver, blood vessels, skin, and psyche— on every single cell. Of course, toxins alone are not the only thing that makes us sick or tired.

Diseases Have Many Causes

The side effects of a sick bowel have a history. There were times when Chinese physicians believed that tones (yes, a musical or vocal sound) made the spleen move, which then tickled the stomach, and, in this way, promoted digestion. Today, we know that the spleen's responsibility is to produce, store, and sort blood cells. It is indeed located next to the stomach, but there's no tickling going on.

Back then, no one even knew that the pancreas existed. They also thought that the right kidney produced sperm. Yet Chinese doctors were very familiar with the functions of the stomach and small and large intestines. They knew how to infer from daily bowel movements the state of their health and could influence bowel movements (and, thereby, the health of their bowels) with precise diet restrictions. At every acupuncture appointment, no matter what the illness was, exact instructions on how and what to eat were an integral part of treatment.

Even farther west, people were convinced that a sick intestine had far-reaching consequences. Hippocrates, the founder of medicine as a science and the most important doctor of ancient times, lived about 2,400 years ago and was sure that "death sits in the bowels" and all diseases begin in the gut.

If we look at the number of annually treated benign and malignant intestinal tumors, diverticula, inflammations, and irritated bowels these days, we can tell that our intestines aren't doing very well. And if the organ that feeds us isn't doing well, we can bet that this has consequences for the whole body.

The human bowel is often compared to the roots of a plant. It's not as far-fetched as it seems—both of them are responsible for taking in nourishment. If a patient has a sick heart, the whole body suffers. The same applies if the kidneys or brain gets sick. These are all pivotal organs whose health plays an essential role when the body gets sick or heals.

The thing that's special about our intestines is that they directly affect the health of our other organs, and it's relatively easy to keep our intestines healthy. Most human diseases are multifactorial, which means that many factors must come together before we get sick. Think of a disease as a whole cake—every piece of cake is one of these factors.

Most illnesses are made of many pieces of a cake in different sizes. There is one factor we have no control over—genetics. What our parents pass down to us is usually just a weakness, a predisposition, or susceptibility, but not an actual sickness. We can't do anything about these preconditions.

Other factors are, for example, infections or the medical condition of a central organ, such as the heart or kidneys. And we can't forget the brain and psyche, which play an important role in almost all diseases. These are all possible factors that, when added together, wear us down increasingly.

Once we finish baking the cake (disease) and all the pieces are together, we get sick. If we take one piece of the cake away, it's often enough to make us feel better. And now comes what you already suspected: if we take out the piece of cake that is the "intestines and nutrition," it's not that difficult to control our health.

Which diseases are affected by the toxins in our intestines? And how do we explain what happens?

The list of diseases that an intestinal regeneration, and the resulting change of the intestinal flora, can cure or significantly alleviate is long.

Arteriosclerosis is a hardening of the arteries. It can lead to heart attacks or strokes. We can easily monitor the effects of this disease, which helps us understand the extent of the damage.

The heart pumps a daily supply of two thousand gallons of blood through our arterial blood vessels and provides our organs and every single cell in our bodies with oxygen, nutrients, and vitamins. The walls of the arteries have three layers. The middle layer consists of muscle fiber and regulates our blood pressure by constricting or dilating the vessels. Leading directly away from the heart, arteries are exceptionally elastic, which is very important in controlling the pressure spikes of the beating heart.

Farther away from the heart, the arteries use the muscles found in the wall's middle layer to create more pressure when necessary, for example when they need to increase the supply of oxygen. In smokers, this muscle layer is inflamed and suffers from degenerative changes, which can result in arteriosclerosis and high blood pressure.

Over one hundred years ago, scientists were already able to demonstrate that *indol* and *phenol*, the toxins derived from putrefaction processes in the intestines, could damage arteries just as much as nicotine. As already described, the liver converts or breaks these poisons down when they are absorbed in small amounts. If a sick intestine allows large amounts to be absorbed into the blood and there are no more detoxification options left, the toxins trigger a reaction in the tissue and also in the blood vessels. The reaction could be a slight, gradual inflammation with nevertheless serious consequences.

If the inflammation is pronounced, our bodies try to protect and close off the area with cholesterol. This is why deposits gather along the vessel walls. It's similar to a scab that builds on a wound and doesn't fall off until everything below it is back to normal. Since the irritation from the toxins doesn't usually stop, the protective layer gets thicker and thicker, and in the worst-case scenario, it entirely closes off the blood vessel. If this happens to an artery near the heart, a heart attack occurs. In all developed countries, cardiovascular diseases are by far the most common cause of death. You've probably read several times that it has something to do with our diet. Now you know why!

The poisonous substances in our bowels that are responsible for silent inflammation (the medical term for the chronic inflammation described above) often make us tired and reduce our ability to concentrate. Many rheumatic diseases are also linked to these toxins, such as thyroid diseases, depression, and other malignant diseases.

The skin is one of the few organs where we can actually see these changes with our naked eyes. Inflammation, eczema, or simply an unhealthy facial color are visible warning signals of possible intestinal toxins—not to mention skin problems can hurt our self-esteem.

A MOODY ORGAN—HOW EMOTIONS INFLUENCE OUR DIGESTION AND OUR INTESTINES INFLUENCE OUR EMOTIONS

For many years, the intestines lived in the shadows in regard to how much media attention they received, only to pop out of nowhere one day to compete against the brain for the spotlight. The public had discovered the "abdominal brain."

For a long time, we thought everything was clear: the brain is the boss; nerves connect the organs and muscles to the brain; and the brain commands what needs to be done. However, the brain can't be all that much of a boss, if some organs can shut down. For example, we can willingly fart, because we control the last and first few centimeters of our digestive system. But when it comes to business in between these regions, and our intestines don't feel like working for whatever reason, our brains have no control.

The Discovery of the Abdominal Brain

In 1862, the German doctor Leopold Auerbach made an amazing discovery. He specialized in pathological changes of the nerves. For this reason, he unrelentingly searched for causes. While looking at a piece of bowel under a microscope, he found a *plexus*, a thick network of nerves of various diameters embedded between two muscle layers. The meaning and purpose of this discovery remained a mystery during his lifetime, yet it received his name, the *Auerbach's plexus*. With one hundred million nerve cells, it is the largest collection of nerves outside of the brain!

This plexus is busy around the clock controlling the movements of the digestive tract, gathering and sharing information about our food from the immune cells, considering hormonal influences, and here and there taking orders from the real boss via detours. It does all this on its own, as the English scientists William Bayliss and Ernest Starling discovered only a few years after Auerbach's death.

They severed an anesthetized dog's nerves that connected the intestines to the brain, so that the brain could only communicate with the body using blood vessels. They wanted to prove that the brain isn't necessary for intestinal activity. Under pressure, the bowel moved in peristaltic waves, pushing the imaginary chyme farther. They injected the same dog with hydrochloric acid in the duodenum in order to simulate a gastric emptying, whereupon the pancreas secreted neutralizing juices, thus proving the bowel's autonomous, self-reliant functioning without the boss. Science had discovered the so-called abdominal brain.

Your Gut Feeling—Just a Bundle of Nerves

In spite of the abdominal brain's autonomy, both of our brains work more closely together than we sometimes want them to. When we're nervous about upcoming exams, we're stuck on the toilet with diarrhea, and if we're traveling, nothing works. If we're constipated, we're in a bad mood; if we're in a bad mood, we're often constipated. Fear makes our stomachs ache. The nerves—or, really, the influence of the autonomic nervous system—are behind all this.

If the digestive tract could do its work entirely independently, anytime day or night, relaxed or tense, it would be great. On the other hand, it would be uneconomical, regarding the available energy for the rest of the body. Maybe that's why the autonomic nervous system (the portion of the brain that we cannot control) gets involved.

To understand this concept, you need to know a little more about that nervous system. The *enteric* (or *intrinsic*) *nervous system* of the digestive tract is one of three divisions of the *autonomic*, or *visceral, ner-*

vous system. It involuntarily regulates our vital functions, such as blood pressure, heartbeat, breathing, metabolism, sexual activity, and, yes, our digestion.

The other two divisions are called the *sympathetic* and *parasympathetic nervous systems.* In contrast, the *somatic* (or *voluntary*) *nervous system* is what we use to govern our conscious reactions.

The sympathetic nervous system once regulated our vital functions, when we were hunting buffalo. These days, it governs when we're stressed out at work or fighting with our neighbors. It prepares us for when we need excessive energy. This procedure affects the intestines as well. They're inhibited by the irritants of the sympathetic nervous system, because energy is needed elsewhere for stressful situations. If stress gets the upper hand, our bowels react with pain, nausea, or frequent belching, because they're no longer up to snuff. The stomach doesn't empty itself, the peristaltic movement is curbed in the small intestine, and only the large intestine becomes more active in some people. In the same way, continuous stress keeps us from properly digesting our food. This can manifest itself as diarrhea or constipation, and cranks up the toxin production in the intestines. The bowel becomes more permeable. The attack of toxins and the triggered defense mechanisms could explain some depressive moods.

The parasympathetic nervous system, on the other hand, controls all functions related to rest and regeneration. Even if the digestive tract has its own nervous system, the parasympathetic nervous system stimulates an increase in digestive juice secretion, better peristalsis, and elimination of our stool—the latter wouldn't have been very practical during buffalo hunting. We wouldn't have slain a single one.

Getting back to the abdominal brain, the intestines regulate and govern a large part of their work using their own nervous system, while the sympathetic and parasympathetic systems intervene with the brain's orders when energy is needed elsewhere.

All this usually happens unconsciously. You'd think that our consciousness would be completely overloaded with all the information our intestines send it. But that's why data doesn't arrive unless something is wrong; for example, when our nerves report pain to the voluntary nervous system.

This is what happens with a lot of people who have an irritable bowel. Their irritant threshold (the threshold that determines when information becomes conscious) is lower. In one study, a researcher blew up a balloon in the intestines of patients with an irritable colon until they felt pain and recorded the patients' brain activity, proving that data arrived increasingly in the section of the brain we call the *limbic system*, unlike what happens in healthy people. Our emotional lives are largely housed in the limbic system; patients who suffer from phobias have increased activity in this area.

After reading the above, you can see that there is a spectrum of irritants that can affect digestion through the autonomic nervous system. And we know from personal experience that not only stress but other strong feelings can upset our stomachs, like love, grief, fear, or fury. By the same token, our intestines influence our well-being, putting us in a state of indigestion, feeling weighed down, or even having a nauseated, "butterflies" feeling in our stomachs.

Because of all this, we can assume that our emotions and digestive tract interact and that our limbic systems communicate with our digestion, as we are now aware that our emotions are housed in the limbic system in the brain, exactly like the information from our intestines.

So we can be pretty sure that a healthy bowel does its part for emotional stability. By the same token, chronic emotional conditions, such as fear or stress, have a negative effect on our digestion. We can do some good for our intestines and overall well-being by trying a therapy that helps us relax and balance our emotions, such as yoga, autogenous training, or meditation.

HELP, MY STOMACH IS GROWING! MY HEART GROANS AND MY SPINAL CORD CRIES

A big belly is annoying and usually the result of gas and bloating. We struggle buttoning up our shirts, and the waistlines of our pants are overly snug. Basically everything is tight except our stomachs. And we eventually get used to this uncomfortable feeling. If it happens suddenly from one day to the next, we may notice the strain, but usually it grows slowly over years until it reaches a critical mass that we've just learned to live with. Now, our bellies may bother us when we exercise or tie our shoes. They may bother us when we have to put on a swimsuit for the beach or when we want to lie on our stomachs. A bloated belly certainly isn't sexy, and who enjoys looking at themselves in the mirror when they have a large gut staring back at them?

There have been times throughout history when society embraced and valued a large belly. It was a sign of wealth, prosperity, and achievement. It was a status symbol, just like a house with a yard and a car. By the time it became the norm and no longer an exception, our understanding of good health had changed. The stomach became the symbol for self-indulgence and loss of control, and a six-pack became our new standard in a body-conscious world.

Most people think that a stomach is the same thing as a huge accumulation of fat. However, fat doesn't have the same consistency in our bodies as a pig stomach at the meat counter. The fat that spans the skin of our stomach is fluid, like warm margarine. We can suck it out!

After it grows only a few centimeters thick, the fat starts hanging and builds an apron. The belly button becomes hard to see since it lies at the end of a long path through a layer of fat. No one is proud to carry around a stomach like that. But really most stomachs are a mixture of blown-up intestinal loops, lymph fluids, and then fat—fat being the smallest part of the bulge.

And a fat stomach doesn't only upset our social lives; it upsets neighboring organs within the body, putting a strain on our overall health. It makes the lungs work harder, the heart groans, there's pressure on the bladder and uterus, and the spinal cord cries from the heavy load.

Other issues caused by a large stomach are the lack of space and inability of the organs to move around. The stomach and chest areas are confined to the space between the pubic bone below and collarbone above. The thorax is protected by the bony rib cage. There is no wiggle room. The diaphragm separates the two regions. Even though the liver is on the right side under the rib cage and the stomach on the left, they are part of the same general "abdominal area." In the breast area, we come across the heart and the lungs. If we need more room in the abdominal area because of an enlarged stomach, a more or less enlarged liver, and gassy, blown-up intestinal loops, it becomes tight in the breast region.

Moaning Lungs

Every day, we inhale about eighteen thousand times and exhale just as often. Our lung volume is 3 to 6 liters (0.8 to 1.6 gallons), if we exhale and inhale entirely. Competitive athletes can achieve 8 liters (2.1 gallons). When we breathe normally, we inhale about .5 liters (1 pint) of air and provide the blood with necessary oxygen, which then reaches every single cell through the bloodstream. The carbon dioxide that accrues in our tissues is transported to the lungs and leaves our bodies as we exhale.

We can inhale thanks to the dome-shaped diaphragm, which sits closely below the two lungs. When it contracts, the lungs are pulled downward, which creates a vacuum, and air flows into the lungs. There are muscles between the ribs that help a little.

We don't need any muscles to exhale. The diaphragm relaxes, and the lungs contract via the *elastic recoil*. The easiest way to imagine this process is to think of a rubber band that springs back to its original shape after it has been stretched.

You can imagine what happens with our breathing if the stomach needs too much room. It hinders inhaling! The diaphragm wants to pull downward, but the upper abdominal organs are pushing upward. The result is shallow breathing with reduced ventilation and oxygen absorption in the lungs. If a doctor x-rayed the breast cavity, she'd write down "elevated diaphragm" in her report, which frequently leads to shortness of breath.

Another drawback to having a large belly is that at night, when we're lying horizontally, the missing gravity (the gravity reduces the upper stomach's size compared to when we're standing) causes extremely bad pressure ratios. This hinders deep breaths of air needed for regeneration in the body and is often the cause of deafening snoring. It's no wonder we wake up sometimes feeling like we haven't slept well, or at all, and find our partners sleeping on the sofa.

The Groaning Heart

The heart is by far one of our favorite organs. One reason is the emotions we ascribe to the heart—even though we clearly feel butterflies in our stomachs when we're in love, no one would ever consider signing a love letter with an image of a stomach or an intestine. On top of that, the heart doesn't have bad breath, it doesn't produce smelly gases, it doesn't have to worry about toxins like the liver, kidneys, and skin do, and it's not stuck in a bony prison like the brain. It beats energetically and happily about one hundred thousand times a day, encased between the two lungs.

The heart doesn't live in a suburban house with a large yard, but rather in an apartment complex with a lot of neighbors. Separated by the diaphragm, the stomach lives right below the heart. The stomach isn't an easygoing neighbor who is happy to rhythmically breathe in and out all day long like the lungs; he's sometimes empty and sometimes full, and when he's not feeling well he stops working for a while, which raises his neighbor's pressure. It's impossible for the heart to avoid interaction with such close neighbors.

Imagine what would happen if your neighbor suddenly claimed 30 percent of your yard. You'd lose your shit, pun intended. Nevertheless, these internal interactions weren't described until 1912 by the German general practitioner Dr. Ludwig Roemheld. He noticed that some patients with severe heart problems had healthy hearts but large upper abdomens, a lot of gas in the intestines, and enlarged stomachs.

The list of symptoms he describes reminds us of a severely sick heart: a tight, heart attack–like feeling in the chest and the related anxiety; shortness of breath or even respiratory distress; strong blood pressure fluctuations; dizziness and hot flashes; pulse fluctuations;

heart palpitations; and nighttime cardiac arrhythmia. As already described above, these symptoms occurred when the patient was lying in a horizontal position and worsened when pressure ratios changed.

These symptoms went down in the books as *gastric cardia* (a complex of gastro-cardiac symptoms), or *Roemheld syndrome*. It is important to know that heart problems may be caused by this syndrome, since the treatment for a constricted heart is entirely different than the treatment for heart problems caused by inadequate blood supply, just like anxiety caused by a constricted heart requires a different therapy than anxiety caused by something else.

The Crying Spinal Cord

In developed countries, almost every other person complains about back problems. In America, back pain is the number-one cause of personal days taken off work. What does the bowel—or, better said, stomach—have to do with it? The stomach influences the positioning of the spine, which changes our posture (see figure on page 77).

Compare your stomach to a fanny pack—you know, the pouches people wrap around their waists to keep small valuables safe during vacation? Obviously, a fanny pack alone won't cause issues with your posture. But imagine it five times bigger and holding a couple of bricks. When a stomach reaches the size of a roller suitcase wrapped around your hips, you can understand the issue.

How we deal with the extra baggage depends on how fit and muscular we are. In order to balance the weight, we either lean forward or backward. For the spinal cord, both possibilities mean that the vertebrae are no longer aligned properly.

If a person suffers from back pain, to figure out if it's caused by the stomach, hug the person from behind and lift up their stomach. If they feel immediate relief from their back pain, the stomach was at least part of the problem.

However, there are more hardships waiting for the spinal cord, like a herniated (slipped) disc! The spinal discs are fibrocartilaginous structures that lie between adjacent vertebrae. The inner gel-like centers have a high water content and act as shock absorbers, cushioning the impact of the body's activities.

If we have bad posture from always leaning forward due to a fat stomach, we increase the pressure on the front side of the spinal discs, and then, similar to when we take a big bite out of a hamburger and the meat slips out, the disc can get squished backward, rupturing the fibro-cartilaginous ring. This causes a slipped disc, which is exceptionally painful and usually squeezes off the running connections in the nerve canal. That explains nerve failure in the legs, bladder, or even intestines.

By the same token, if we have bad posture from always leaning back, something similar happens, but with pressure on the back side of the spinal discs. These slipped discs don't cause nerve failure, though,

POOR POSTURE DIAGRAM

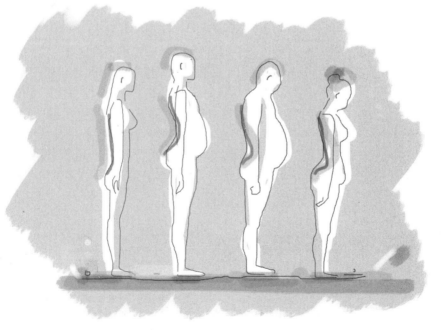

Correct Posture   Poor Posture Related to
                         Stomach Size

because there are limited bundles of nerve fibers on the front sides. This anterior disc herniation is less common, although equally painful.

A much more common disorder resulting from poor posture is vertebral blockage, which can cause low back pain (lumbago). Poor posture often comes from a combination of bad positioning of the spine and very few back muscles that also could prevent a blockage. Even if we had more muscles, people often balance out a bigger stomach with poor posture.

Exercise programs that claim they'll give you a flat stomach are a dime a dozen. Unfortunately, few of them address the root of the problem—bloat caused by blown-up intestinal loops and gas. We can strengthen our stomach muscles, which is a good idea in general, and with a strong musculature, we can suck in our stomachs all day long to create the illusion of a flat stomach, but that sure gets old fast. These quick flat-stomach programs often get poor results as well because they ignore the importance of strengthening the back muscles. But when it comes to a bulging belly, the biggest culprit is an unhealthy gut.

As a reminder, a big stomach is not only a well-fed potbelly where the many calories find their home; instead, the stored-up fat is actually one of the smallest factors at play. To truly address a protruding belly we also must change how the gut is functioning. We can reduce, for example, our gas production by participating in a training program specifically for the intestines, changing our eating habits permanently, and choosing the right foods. We can also prevent the production of toxins that wear out our intestines. And in this way, we'll be on our way to a flat stomach and healthy life.

ANNA, MAX, AND PAULA GET THEIR CRAP TOGETHER

By now, you might have realized that the health problems that have been bugging you for some time may be caused by your digestion, which isn't quite up to par. You are probably also aware of what you do to contribute to this.

A few real-life examples can provide a more in-depth look at the connections between our overall health and the bowel. It is impossible to trace all problems back to a sick intestine, but more often than you think, it is at least a part of the cause.

For Anna and Max, eating habits play a decisive role in their poor health. Then there's Paula, who belongs to an early generation that had to make food stretch. She kept this moderate eating style as a life-long habit, which proved healthy and beneficial, as her story will show. Unfortunately, many others in Paula's generation had a hard time maintaining balanced diets when most foods became available in almost unlimited quantities,.

Anna

It was vacation time again, the best time of the year—the time for catching a few rays in peace, enjoying delicious food and drink, reading, or simply chilling for a few hours (something her children seemed particularly good at). Anna knew what to expect. She had bought the little house in Provence some years ago, when it became clear that moving from hotel to hotel throughout the summer could not provide her with the relaxation she needed. All she wanted now, though, was to put the first five days behind her! Bowel movements, if she had them at all, were torture. Nothing helped. In the past, when they'd stayed in hotels, she had put it down to the unfamiliar toilets. In their house in Provence, they had tried to create an atmosphere similar to the one at home, but it hadn't made much difference. She had tried everything: drinking plenty of water, taking laxatives in varying quality and quantity—all a complete waste of time. And although everything was pretty much trouble-free at home, she suspected something had been wrong with her bowels for some time.

Toward the end of her second pregnancy, she had discovered what hemorrhoids felt like. She couldn't remember having had bowel problems in her childhood. Maybe she hadn't had a daily bowel movement, but it hadn't bothered her. She could, however, remember her belly, which she'd always found too big. She would've happily done without it.

It was true that she wasn't particularly athletic, but exercise was important to her, so she did yoga and Pilates a few hours a week, which left her more or less satisfied with her figure. But it made no difference to her belly. She could, of course, suck it in if she felt someone looking at her, but that was not a long-term solution.

She had also had back problems for what felt like forever. A slipped disc two years ago had prevented her from doing all kinds of activities, so she had gained weight.

For about six months, her joints had also been giving her trouble. Her hands felt stiff when she woke in the mornings; at other times, it was her shoulders or knees that acted up. She often found herself breaking into a sweat. There was nothing wrong with her hormones, her gynecologist assured her. It wasn't menopause. But knowing that didn't help her any.

She had read in a magazine that normal digestion takes about eighteen hours. The spinach she had eaten at lunch should have colored her stool green the next morning, but it hadn't. If she was lucky, it might happen a day later.

And then there was that other thing. She loved a glass of red wine in the evenings, when the children were finally asleep and the day was over, just to relax. In Provence, of course, she didn't always leave it at the one glass; after all, she was on vacation, and there was nothing wrong with that.

It was Celine, a good friend of hers, who pointed it out to her. "Your teeth are all red," she said. "Have you been watching too many vampire films lately?" Anna wasn't particularly amused. Maybe lipstick, she thought, but the next time she went to the bathroom, she saw that the wine had stained her teeth red, as if her mouth could no longer be bothered to clean itself.

The doctor sent her for a colonoscopy, and apart from the liter of unappetizing liquid she had to drink, it wasn't too horrible. The diagnosis: colon transversum prolongatum. In English, that's an elongated transverse colon, but otherwise, she was fine. That didn't get Anna anywhere, though, because she didn't feel like she was fine.

She thought of her father, who had battled bowel cancer for years before he died two years ago.

And she thought of her husband, who'd been nagging her for years about her eating habits: "Don't wolf your food down like that." She thought of her job, her children—she simply didn't have the time to chew her food thoroughly. That, at any rate, was what she'd been telling herself all these years. But what if her husband was right? He chewed his food properly, and you could hardly smell a thing when he went to the bathroom. His teeth didn't turn red when he drank red wine. He didn't have a potbelly. He had no back problems.

A friend told her about a bowel fitness program. She had had similar issues, and she had begun to improve immediately.

Anna looked into it and decided to start a thorough, professionally supervised program right away—it was time to make a serious effort. And lo and behold, the bowel program left Anna feeling like a new person. She had daily bowel movements; her back trouble almost entirely disappeared; her joints were fully mobile again. It was a clear sign, and Anna took it seriously. She changed her eating habits and improved her quality of life.

Max

Max was a workaholic and always had been. He couldn't imagine a life without work, the ups and downs, the switch from tension to relaxation, and that great feeling of having everything under control.

If he hadn't taken over the family business, he would've ended up in management in the corporate world and had everything under control there. He didn't need much sleep. If he was wide awake at five in the morning, he didn't care; he used the extra hours to get ready for the day. Four to five hours of sleep was enough for him. Under his management, the company flourished; everyone knew that. Yes, you could say he was successful.

At home, too, he had good days and bad days, but not more than anyone else. His children were healthy, and if all went well, his eldest son could soon start working in the company.

The only occasional cause for concern was his health, not that he'd paid a lot of attention to it so far. It was one thing he did not have under control. He had always taken his health for granted.

In his youth, he had been athletic, and in sports he had also been successful. He was convinced the soccer team would have won a lot less without him. Eight years ago, he'd joined the executive board of the soccer club. Since then, he hadn't played any sports; he didn't have the time.

He did, however, notice that his belly was growing bigger and bigger. It began to get in the way; tying his shoelaces got trickier and trickier.

He went to the toilet with Swiss punctuality, at the same time every morning. That must have meant his bowels were healthy—at least, that's what he thought. Although he did leave the toilet in an unbearable state afterward; it had always been that way.

It all started with high blood pressure. He didn't like taking pills, but a man's gotta do what a man's gotta do. Then his heart started acting up; he had palpitations at night. That frightened him a little. He was told he suffered from Roemheld syndrome, which meant that excess gas from his intestinal tract was putting pressure on his heart. He wondered how there could possibly be enough gas left to put pressure on his heart, considering the amount his colon emitted every day. But there were pills for that too.

Maybe it was time to do something about his belly. But that would mean changing his diet, and he really didn't feel like doing that. He liked eating, not that he took his time savoring it; he had no time for that. By the time he finished his meal, others hadn't even eaten half of their own. *Work fast, eat fast* was his motto. His grandmother had taught him that. Slow eaters go nowhere in life. He also liked drinking milk, often as much as half a liter a day.

His bowel made itself known with terrible pains in his left groin. He didn't have time for that at all. Then there was the colonoscopy, and a few polyps were removed and examined.

Luckily nothing malignant, Max was told. He felt reassured.

To prevent the inflammation of the diverticula which had been causing the pain, he was prescribed yet more pills. But the inflammation could still come back, he was told. If that happened, it would be advisable to have part of his colon removed. That got him worried. It was clearly time to deal with his bowels, he decided.

With a thoroughness that was typical of how he approached things, Max made up his mind to do something about his colon. He wanted an established method, no unproven trends. After researching it and asking the advice of his GP, he decided on a regeneration method that the GP himself could carry out. Max thought it looked pretty good.

Every morning—intestinal saline rinses with Epsom salts, chewing training with several-day-old spelt rolls accompanied by a shot glass of root juice (carrot juice for example), and a little soy yogurt. Every evening—tea. His belly was rhythmically massaged every day. That took some time getting used to! But after a few days, he noticed that it was considerably easier for him to tie his shoelaces. The feeling of tension in his abdomen subsided, his heart seemed happy, and his blood pressure returned to normal. After a week, he was healthy enought to start coming off all medications.

A breath test revealed that he had lactose intolerance, so he gave up drinking milk entirely.

After a year, he repeated the program to stabilize the results. Five years after the initial regeneration program, the inflammation has not recurred. His bowel movements are as regular as ever, but now the toilet is usable afterward. His blood pressure is normal without any pills.

He did, however, have to make thorough changes to his eating habits, and he goes without certain foods that he had never thought might be responsible for the state of his health.

Paula

When the Second World War broke out, Paula was just six years old. She can remember what she ate back then, simply because food was something she couldn't take for granted. By today's standards there wasn't much to eat. But Paula almost always had enough and knew that many others were worse off than her. She remembers, too, the ration stamps

issued right from the beginning of the war. At first you could buy vegetables and potatoes. Her aunt who lived in the country helped provide
food for the family as well as she could.

Everything else was rationed; things weren't always available, and
even if they were, there wasn't usually enough money for them. A big
loaf of bread, a pound of meat (the potential ration grew smaller and
smaller as the war progressed), and less than half a pound of fat a week
was the maximum per person, but you never got that much. Her father
ate most of their meat; he had to work hard.

The meager diet, however, had an impact on people's eating habits.
People savored their meals. That meant that people sat at the table longer, chewed more, and made the most of their food. A snack between
meals or a bar of chocolate in a coffee shop wasn't even an option.

Back then, everyone knew that chewing was healthy, and health was
seen as a major asset. That has stayed with Paula all her life.

The main meal was usually eaten at midday. In the evenings, they
ate soup—every kind imaginable. That, too, is a habit that Paula has
largely stuck to.

Of course, they occasionally indulged. But such occasions remained
exceptions. In the fifties, Paula married, and before her daughter was
born, she and her husband left town to go and live in the country.

This made no difference in her eating habits. It was then, when
she was a little over twenty, that she tasted sweet things for the first
time. She hadn't had cake or chocolate before. She loved drinking water;
industrially produced drinks had always been too sweet for her, and in
the summer, she liked making lemonade for her family. Over the years,
she got into the habit of drinking the odd glass of wine in the evening.
At family celebrations she would, of course, have more than just one.
But a lack of moderation was very rare for Paula.

Paula has never been seriously ill, just the odd cold. And ten years
ago, she tore her cruciate ligament skiing. It was the only operation she
has ever had, the only time she has ever seen the inside of a hospital.

She is horrified at the way her grandchildren eat. Cooking seems to have gone out of fashion—she often wonders how it can possibly end well.

In Numbers—The Intestines, and Diseases Caused by Unhealthy Intestines

Number of intestinal bacteria living in your gut—**100 Trillion**
Number of people living on earth—**7 Billion**
Number of Google searches for the word
  "intestines"—**23,000,000**
New cases of colon cancer per 100,000 male residents in the
  United States (2012)—**43**
New cases of colon cancer per 100,000 male residents in
  Western Africa (2012)—**5**
Dietary fiber intake in the United States (grams per day)—**16**
Dietary fiber intake in Western Africa (grams per day)—**30**
Ambulatory care visits due to diverticular disease in the United
  States (2004)—**3,200,000**
Treatments for diverticulitis per year in Western Africa—**Rare**
Americans affected by gastrointestinal disease each year—
  70,000,000
Americans affected by chronic constipation (2000)—
  63,000,000
Americans affected by irritable bowel syndrome (estimated)—
  25,000,00–45,000,000
Number of Americans who die of heart disease every year—
  610,000
Percentage of adults in the US with low back pain (2015)—
  29.1%

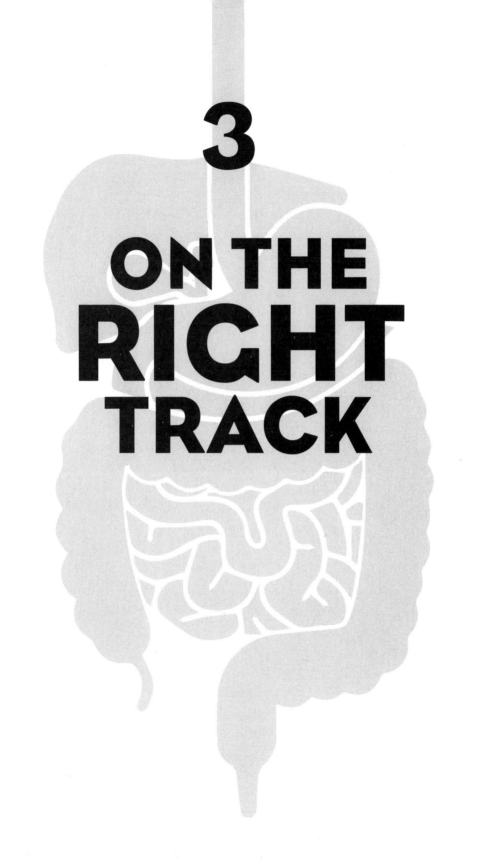

3

ON THE RIGHT TRACK

A FITNESS PROGRAM FOR YOUR INTESTINES

When we think of a fitness program, we associate it with sweaty and difficult activities as well as the motivation it takes to get started. We might have to get up earlier and look for a specialized studio or club where we can sign up for classes that only occur at designated times. In other words, we need to dedicate plenty of time, strength, and energy to improving our health so we can feel better in the end. If we're trying to improve our muscle mass, it's probably the right way to go. But on certain days, we rest because our muscles need to stretch and recover.

If we did the same thing for our bowels, a comparable fitness program would consist of irritating foods that are difficult to digest. In order to give them a good workout, we'd poorly chew massive amounts of sauerkraut morning, noon, and night, and then sit on the toilet for hours. That's pretty idiotic!

Though they are difficult to digest, insufficiently chewed dried fruits are often eaten in the hopes of helping the flagging intestine to get back on its feet again. Similarly, bulking agents, such as psyllium, flax, and chia seeds, are also often used to get the old bowel working again. These strategies work for a while, but eventually we'll have to reach for the laxatives.

Still not getting it? Picture this: You're driving a tired old donkey through the prairie, hoping it suddenly becomes strong and capable again. Wishful thinking.

We need an entirely different program for our intestines, because they need rest to get fit and regenerate. They are like a broken bone that has to be held in place until it's strong again. Nobody would run a marathon right after breaking his or her leg.

Our bowels are usually overworked by colossal meals that we scarf down, snacks that don't give our bowels the chance to clean themselves, and abundant dinners that don't give a minute's rest during the regeneration phase.

Furthermore, our intestines suffer from the consumption of industrially modified food that doesn't match our natural nourishment patterns or from eating too much of one type of food that normally doesn't present a problem when consumed in smaller portions. We need to stop eating some foods and take a break from others to help our bowels feel good again. It's all about breaking bad habits and changing them for the long term. This is just as hard, if not harder, than going to the gym for some people.

For a healthy gut, we must also influence and change the intestinal flora, since it's mostly responsible for diseases caused by the production of bacterial toxins in a sick bowel. Anything that makes our guts healthier helps the intestinal flora as well.

Shortly, I will introduce the tools that proved effective during my years treating thousands of people with these very issues. The basic program lasts a mere ten days, a manageable timeframe. During this time, you'll either maintain or improve the performance of your intestines; you'll clean and detoxify them. The program is also about paying close attention to your eating behavior and then, if necessary, changing it and practicing new behavior.

It is a modern detox program that targets our intestines and, therefore, our entire health.

At first, you'll need to make small changes for a week leading up to the program's start. Later, you'll attempt to apply what you learned to eating a healthy diet. Overall, your intestines will be the center of attention for three weeks. Your health will thank you for it. I'll show you how you can solidify the new treatment of your intestines with regular training days.

This program is preventive. If you have any health disorders, I advise you to do the program under professional supervision and to plan on spending more time on it. You can find a list of the specially trained therapists at the International Society of Mayr Physicians (the info is provided in the selected bibliography and resources in the back of the book, page 160).

There is one small problem with this fitness program: it makes you addicted! Once you experience how you feel with a healthier bowel, you'll want the same experience again and again. It does, however, depend on what kind of person you are when dealing with your health and regeneration.

But first, let's look at the necessary background knowledge, so that the ten-day program is as easy as pie!

CONSERVATION IS KEY— THE GENTLE WAY TO FAST

Gandhi fasted—no surprise there. But so do Julia Roberts, Will Smith, Liv Tyler, Ben Affleck, and Beyoncé. I could fill up this book with a list of famous actors and performers who fast to shed pounds quickly. Even if the reasons for fasting are as different as the people doing it, the positive results for our minds and bodies are the same. Fasting is at the forefront of the things in life that we know are healthy and life prolonging.

Overweight binge eaters often try to convince us that fasting isn't healthy or is even dangerous. They probably just can't imagine life without their favorite pastime. But it's actually not that hard, and the period following the fast is like fireworks for your taste buds, sense of smell, and every single cell.

Fasting is very human. Animals, though, cannot fast; they starve when they have nothing to eat. The personal decision to stop eating for a while is reserved for humans alone. Starving is not a way to heal for humans, either. Starving is a consequence if we can't find food, and it always comes with a feeling of panic, which triggers a vegetative reaction that negatively influences our organs. After starving for two to three days, we enter a life-threatening situation.

The decisive difference with fasting is that we voluntarily do without certain solids or liquids. But don't worry. As you'll soon see, there are ways to reach the same goal with less abstinence.

The leaders of the mainstream religions (Buddha, Jesus, Mohammed) were all for fasting, because the body and mind grow stronger and more resilient. Without exception, the most famous doctors and philosophers (Theophrastus, Galenus, Hippocrates) recommended fasting, even if they didn't all agree on the timing.

What happens to our bodies when we fast? How do we explain the positive effect it has on our health?

Attempts at explaining these effects began with Clive McCay's research in 1935. He was able to show that rats lived almost twice as long if they received very little to eat for a while. He didn't stop feeding the rats completely, because it's not possible with animals, as already mentioned.

Since then, there have been numerous hypotheses about the reason for this effect on the rats. A few years ago, Valter Longo, an Italian American biogerontologist and cell biologist, demonstrated that reducing the intake of food decreases a substance in our bodies called insulin-like growth factor 1 (IGF-1). The level of this substance is high in a protein-rich, overabundant diet (widespread in developed countries these days) and decreases when we fast or eat less.

People who cannot produce this protein due to a hereditary disease suffer from Laron's syndrome. It causes short stature and oftentimes obesity, but also prevents the patient from getting cancer or cardiovascular diseases. In a mountain range in Ecuador, about 130 people live with this genetic defect. Healthy nutrition isn't even an issue for them, since they are immune to most of our lifestyle diseases.

If the IGF-1 level in our blood is high, it affects growth and rapid cell division. If it is low, our bodies go back to regenerating and repairing damaged cells, and that's already half the battle when dealing with our health.

From the moment we are born, our cells start the process of being damaged around fifty thousand times a day. That's every single cell in our bodies. But our bodies are amazing, and those damaged cells simply repair themselves—that is, until we reach a certain age and that ability is impaired. A recent study by German professor Jörg Bergemann showed that individuals with low DNA repair capacity can restore this cellular healing ability to a regular state after ten days of calorie reduction. A normal DNA repair capacity contributes to healthier aging.

It has also been proven that, when calorie intake levels are low, normal cells are protected from the toxicity during chemotherapy, but cancerous cells aren't. That is a promising beginning for the treatment of malignant diseases.

What happens to our intestines when we fast or drastically reduce our food intake? Toxins in our food are no longer absorbed and are no longer produced in our colons. In other words, we take away our intestinal germs' food; or rather, we reduce the bad bacteria and strengthen the good ones. The intestines have a lot of free time, and after a couple of days, so do all our detoxification organs: the liver, lungs, skin, and kidneys. Since they don't have a lot to do anymore, noticeable energy is released. However, during this time, our overall endurance is low.

The Right Diet While Fasting

Which diet is best when fasting or when eating reduced amounts of food? Since eating very little has been scientifically proven to be effective, eating nothing would be a hard, unnecessary path to take. As you will discover, there's a gentler way.

In the past, there have been many successful experiments to spare the intestines and positively influence the intestinal flora by eating less. The Swiss physiologist Emil Abderhalden recommended milk when the human digestive tract was no longer able to digest raw produce. In 1866, Philipp Karell, the personal physician of Tzar Nicholas I, published an article about milk cures that he successfully implemented over two decades. John Harvey Kellog practiced chewing cornflakes with his patients and gave them milk to supply them with nutrients and influence their intestinal flora. If you are familiar with today's Kellogg's

Corn Flakes, you have to be asking yourself how anyone could train in chewing it. Well, the consistency has clearly changed over the years.

For Dr. Franz Xaver Mayr, a diet consisting of milk and bread rolls was an integral part of his therapy for many years. In his 1920 book, Die Darmträgheit (*The Sluggishness of the Bowel*), he wrote, "This milk-bread diet has to reluctantly accept the argument that it isn't nutritious enough for us, because the donors—cows—cannot eat what nature intended and, chained to a feeding trough in gloomy, barely ventilated, dark stalls, have to lead a highly unhealthy life."

To avoid any confusion, I'd like to interject that even back then, it wasn't always easy to obtain high-quality milk. Dr. Mayr placed a lot of importance on the quality of the milk. It couldn't be pasteurized and had to come from grazing cows with small udders.

These diets have remained popular over the years because of their positive effects. The milk and its nutrients are almost completely absorbed in the first half of the small intestine, which means the rest of the small intestine and the entire large intestine have more or less nothing to do. The complete absorption of these proteins and nutrients swallowed in the milk makes way for an almost entirely free large intestine. There is nothing left to trigger putrefaction, and the body, therefore, receives a break from the byproducts of digestion. This means that the stressful toxins disappear.

If some of the germs in the milk make it through the gastric acid in the stomach, they can find their way intact through the small intestine and change the intestinal flora. Like the gastric acids, homogenization or pasteurization destroys these germs, too, but through heat or chemical treatments. The spores make it through these treatments because they are very resistant. They reach the large intestine and crank up the putrefaction processes.

Today's milk, as well as our knowledge about the negative effects of lactose intolerance and the adverse impact of milk proteins if they are consumed in large quantities, has discredited these milk diets along with the idea of chewing cornflakes or white bread rolls to improve our chewing muscles. Today's bread rolls have three times more gluten content than before, and the protein component ATI, which is used as an insecticide, causes digestion problems for some. Bread made of spelt flour could still be used to practice chewing.

As with any diet you undertake to improve the health of your bowel, it's important you let your digestive tract rest during the program; you need to give it a lot of free time. Additionally, you should always pay attention to what you can tolerate. Since everyone's digestive tract is so different based on its condition and performance, it's impossible to create a standard formula for everybody.

You should always follow some basics:

As gentle as possible! This depends on your physique, overall health, and spare time. For example, if you have time to obtain raw milk from healthy cows with small udders, you could consume milk during the gentle phase of the program, as long as you don't have a milk allergy and aren't lactose intolerant. You could also consume yogurt made from unhomogenized milk, organic soy yogurt, or coconut milk yogurt. Small amounts of freshly juiced root vegetables, such as carrots, celery, and red beets, as well as equally small amounts of green smoothies, are ideal for providing all the vital substances you need during the program. Almond milk or other nut drinks also contain enough nutrients to supply you with what you'll need.

In order to treat your intestines gently, proper chewing is a must. To practice chewing and, at the same time, gain the right feeling of fullness, dry spelt bread, dry gluten-free bread, or all kinds of nuts work well. Coconut chips or fresh coconuts are especially suitable, as they contain monolauric acid, a fatty acid that has antiviral and antibacterial attributes and can be found in mother's milk.

As fiber-free as possible! Fiber is indispensable for a healthily functioning bowel. But that's not true during the gentle phase! While you're letting your intestines rest, you should stay away from fiber, because it takes away the colon's free time. Your colon has to work hard to pass on the undigested fibers.

The harder to digest, the more you need to chew! If you can't follow a strict diet to give your intestines a break, you should try to exaggeratedly chew your food, like Horace Fletcher did, to achieve maximum bowel rest. He chewed each bite one hundred times; his meal consisted of thirty bites.

Strict fasting in the evening! Dinners put a lot of strain on our bowels, but sometimes they're hard to avoid, whether they be work related or for a cozy evening at home with friends. But you have to do without during the gentle phase! This way, you can give your intestines eighteen hours between lunch and breakfast the next day to cleanse themselves and regenerate. It also keeps your calorie counts down, which helps you feel the positive effects of the fasting. This has to be the hardest part for many. The first two or three days, your body misses that evening meal it was so used to over the years, but these days go by fast. The fact that you'll feel so much better compensates for the missed meals.

F. X. Mayr

Over a hundred years ago, an Austrian doctor made waves. Dr. Franz Xaver Mayr, the bowel specialist, was more fascinated with the digestive tract than anyone else. Not that there aren't any doctors these days who are fascinated with the digestive tract, but when today's doctors dedicate their time to this organ, it's usually just one section of it. They become, for example, fixated on the anus or stomach, or they're looking at large intestines all day long.

Franz Xaver Mayr was born in the town of Gröbming, Austria, in 1875. He studied medicine at the University of Graz and, during practical training, came into contact with patients suffering from severe digestive disorders. After prescribing them bland diets and daily stomach treatments that unblocked the abdominal area and activated the intestinal muscles, he noticed that their digestive problems improved, as did parallel symptoms that didn't appear to have anything to do with the intestinal issues.

Inspired by his experience, he began to learn everything he could about the intestines. He noticed that one could determine the health of every other human organ, like the heart or kidney, based solely on its size. So one question he asked himself was why this wasn't possible for the intestines as well.

He graduated in 1901 and began to work in the famous spa town of Carlsbad in 1906. Encouraged by his studies and treatments, he wrote down the guidelines for an optimally healthy digestive tract. He wrote about the interaction between the different digestive parts and their effects on the surrounding organs as well as the entire body. He did all this with a degree of precision that had not existed before.

From then on, digestive disorders could be determined by measuring the abdomen and palpating the digestive tract. Poor posture of the spinal cord could be traced back to certain digestive disorders and then remedied. In his book *Die Darmträgheit* (*The Sluggishness of the Bowel*), he described these connections in layman's terms and made the "basics of digestive diseases" easy to read for the general public.

Letting the digestive tract rest was of primary importance in his treatments. He recommended all kinds of diets, from fasting to bland home cooking, depending on the patient's tolerance and his or her disorder. At the same time, he'd rinse out and treat the intestines with diluted Espon salts every day, so they could regenerate. That's how the Mayr cure eventually became a widely accepted naturopathic therapy.

Mayr held seminars at the Charité Universitätsmedizin Berlin (a large teaching hospital in Berlin) and the Mayo Clinic. Much later in life, he also founded the International Society of Mayr Physicians, which today has approximately six hundred members worldwide.

CLEAN, CLEANER, CLEANEST—
SPRING CLEANING FOR YOUR INTESTINES

At times, the concept of cleaning our intestines has worried some doctors. To make things perfectly clear, our intestines can do it best by themselves. After all, we're dealing with about three thousand square feet. Even if we could take a steam jet down there, it would take us at least half a day or longer. And since we can assume that rinsing the bowel like that would only *clean* the sick intestinal mucosa and not *regenerate* it, everything would go back to the way it was in one or two days.

Have you ever had a sick mouth mucosa? After a meal, the mouth cannot clean itself like it normally does, and leftover food remains behind. You could simply rinse it down with a glass of water, but you'd just have the same problem after the next meal. The mouth cannot clean itself until the mucosa is healthy again. So anything we try with the bowel mucosa may, at best, help *support* regeneration and, hence, the bowel's ability to clean itself.

When it comes to rinsing, we only have two options: from the top down or from the bottom up. From the bottom up, an enema, is not everyone's thing, but it is the oldest method to rid the colon of built-up stool. We can find this method in Egyptian, Greek, and Indian medicine and probably in all the cultures of the world. The goal was and is always to give the intestines a short break, whether before an operation or because of chronic constipation. The enema only reaches the large intestine. The small intestine cannot be rinsed this way. As mentioned earlier, there is a valve between the small and large intestines that blocks a rinse from this direction. The surface of the large intestine is quite small compared to the small intestine, with all its wrinkles and villi. Plus, the large intestine, even though it's much dirtier, spends a lot less time absorbing toxins. Therefore, rinsing from the bottom up is only of limited use.

Epsom Salts

You can, however, rinse from the top down. We could try it with large amounts of water. Admittedly, this would be fatal, because the intestines would absorb all the water, the volume of blood would increase, and the circulatory system would be overloaded, possibly leading to death by heart failure.

It's different if you use saline water for the rinse. Water with Epsom salts and water with Glauber salts are the most well-known mixtures. These liquids are found in natural springs of cure towns, such as Carlsbad, Teplitz, and Montecanti, that people with digestive disorders often visit. The guests at these spas drink salt water daily, and with good reason. It irrigates the digestive tract gently, depending on the dose.

You probably know of Epsom and Glauber salts as laxatives. You drink a glass, and during the next hours, you're stuck on the toilet while a bucket of water leaves your body. As always, the dosage is key for this effect.

If you were to drink the right dose of saline water as a laxative for only ten days, your intestines wouldn't be any fitter than they were before. On the contrary, they would probably lose strength and energy. As is the case with many laxatives, the intestines lose water as well as potassium, which is important for muscle contractions. The muscles become increasingly weaker, which is why the bowel continues to need laxatives in order to function properly. In the end, the gut becomes addicted to them. If, in daily life, we need a laxative for stubborn constipation, the dosage should be high at first, but then rapidly reduced.

The chemical name for Epsom salts is *magnesium sulfate*, and for Glauber salts, *sodium sulfate*. The sulfate in all saline solutions is responsible for the main effect. The sodium in Glauber salts can lead to increased blood pressure when taken for longer periods of time. Epsom salts don't have this side effect; for this reason, you should give Epsom salts preference.

The bowel cannot absorb sulfate very well, so it sticks to the walls, inhibiting absorption of the water part of the saline solution. Not only is the water poorly absorbed, but the colon's bacterial toxins aren't absorbed as well either—this is a welcome effect.

Unfortunately, the absorption of prescribed medication is also more complicated. Therefore, any prescribed medications must be taken at least thirty minutes before or a few hours after drinking the saline solution.

With the right dosage, the amount of eliminated mushy or liquid stool should be about the same amount as the glass of Epsom salts you drank. If you use concentrations of Epsom salts as a laxative, there will be a lot of sulfate in the intestines. The bowel then tries to dilute it by allowing water to flow in from the body, which explains the laxative effect in high doses.

In the right dosage, Epsom salts lead to an increase in hydrochloric acid in the stomach when there is too little and a decrease in gastric acids when there is too much. The right dosage also triggers secretion in the liver, and the flow of bile is reinforced with neutralizing, high-alkaline content, the counterpart of acid. The bile leads to better movements in the small intestine and, in this way, supports the rinsing effect. Laxative concentrations, on the other hand, trigger the gallbladder to contract in a cramp-like way. If you had gallstones, you'd be painfully aware of a bilious attack. This explains why you should avoid drinking laxative concentrations of saline solutions.

With the right dosage, you may have a bowel movement in one or two hours. This is called a *reflexive bowel movement*. When you have to go to the toilet right after drinking a cup of coffee in the morning, then you've had a reflexive bowel movement. When the stomach is stimulated a little, the large intestine receives this information and empties itself to be on the safe side. In other words, when something is coming from above, it makes room for it just in case. When this happens with Epsom salt solution, you don't eliminate the Epsom salts you just drank, but rather the solution you drank the day before. You'll usually have a bowel movement about four to twelve hours later, and with the right dose, it should have a mushy consistency. All the positive effects listed above are strongest when you drink the saline solution in the morning, on an empty stomach.

Some critics say that the intestinal flora suffers when you use Epsom salts for a long time. But as previously explained, we can easily do without a large portion of our intestinal residents. Research has shown that even after weeks of ingesting this saline solution, a thinned out, harmless intestinal flora still exists.

When used for a long period, you should definitely avoid laxative concentrations of five to six grams or more of Epsom salts. The maximum amount is three grams, which is about one level teaspoon. A heaping teaspoon is already too much.

You buy Epsom salts in crystallized form. The salt has to be stirred into a glass of warm water until you can no longer see the crystals. Cold water stimulates the intestinal peristalsis (wavelike contractions), which is why it is gentler on the bowels if you drink lukewarm to warm water.

Base or Acid? Both!

A balanced acid-base environment is a prerequisite for all metabolic procedures in our bodies. Hyperacidity in the tissue is linked to most lifestyle diseases like high blood pressure, strokes, cancer, and diabetes, as well as muscle and joint diseases—like osteoporosis—and some skin diseases.

Processes in our bodies, whether constructive or destructive in nature, are dependent on a specific environment. If it isn't maintained, there is not enough production or breaking down of substances, which leads to partially toxic intermediate products. These cannot be entirely broken down, thus harming the surrounding tissue. The acid-base balance plays the most important role in securing this environment. How does it do this?

Acids have a corrosive effect, a sour taste, and are familiar to us in acids like acetic acid, hydrochloric acid, or lactic acid. Bases are alkaline and are, to some extent, the counterpart to acids. They are able to neu-tralize acids.

The pH of something is the measure of the acidity or alkalinity of water-soluble substances, where 0 is very acidic and 14 is very basic.

Our blood has a consistent pH value of 7.4. We refer to values under 7.36 as *acidosis*, a.k.a. hyperacidity, and values over 7.44 as *alkalosis*, meaning the blood is then too basic. Deviations below 6.8 and above 7.7 lead to death.

To give you a better idea about pH values, here is a list of different drinks and products along with their pH value:

> Lemon juice: 2.5
> Cola: 2.5
> Wine: 4.0
> Coffee: 5.0
> Milk: 6.5
> Mineral water: 6–7
> Soap: 9.5
> Lye: 13.5

If you imagine these tastes, you'd be surprised to learn that lemon juice and cola are equally acidic. It just doesn't taste like it because cola contains 10 percent sugar. The sour taste is covered by the sugar.

How does a healthy body manage to keep its blood's pH value between 7.36 and 7.44? It has a lot of buffer systems at its disposal to compensate for excessive acids or bases. The blood has some buffer systems as well, and when it needs help to eliminate acids, the lungs, kidneys, skin, and intestines support the blood.

If the buffer systems are overworked for a long period of time, there is increased acidity in other body tissue first, since the top priority is to keep the pH value of the blood under control. More acids must be elim-inated, something you can notice with the kidneys based on the sour smell of your urine and with your skin based on an excessive amount of sour sweat that makes you smell like grapefruit.

Acid-producing fermentation processes in our intestines upset this balance just as much as the excessively acidic foods we eat, like meat, fish, wheat, eggs, and acidic drinks (like sodas and many other sweetened beverages). We can eliminate surplus acids by sweating more while exercising or in the sauna.

In the intestines, you can lessen the fermentation process by not eating huge amounts of fruit, and by avoiding fructose or lactose when you have an intolerance. With alkaline produce, such as nuts, vegetables, and small amounts of ripe fruit, you can have a positive impact on the acid-base environment.

Another way to free your body of acids is really simple: drink water! Just one sip of water already thins out the hydrochloric acid in your stomach. The stomach is designed to balance itself out, so it produces parietal cells, which secrete hydrochloric acid to maintain an acidic environment. At the same time, your stomach produces bicarbonate, a strong base, and passes it on to the blood, where it remains available as a bicarbonate buffer. These are, like so many in our bodies, very complex procedures that are not always easy to understand.

During your fitness program for the bowel, you can strengthen these effects by adding an alkaline powder to your water one to three times a day. Alkaline powders consist mostly of bicarbonate. The alkaline water can neutralize larger amount of acids and, in this way, crank up the bicarbonate production in your stomach.

Drink!

Drinking too little is linked to colon and bladder cancer as well as kidney stones, cardiovascular diseases, and diabetes. When you drink too little, you can't concentrate as well; some people get a headache, and others become constipated. But why is drinking so important? Why does it seem so difficult to pinpoint the right amount of liquids, and how does the liquid we drink cleanse us?

A large part of our bodies, about 50 to 60 percent, consists of water. For a 165-pound man, this would mean he is made of about eleven gallons of water. Every day, about three quarts of that, so 5 to 10 percent, are replenished. If you were to stop drinking water today, you would soon get a headache, and then become tired, and in two days, at the most, you'd collapse. You wouldn't survive much longer than that; whereas, if you voluntarily deprive yourself of food, your body can last thirty days or more.

We have to drink because of four organs. The largest amount of water lost is in our urine, normally 1.6 quarts per day. Right about now, you're probably asking yourself how all that water reaches your bladder in order to be eliminated. Just like the water in food, the water we drink enters the small intestine, where it gets absorbed into the bloodstream. In this way, the volume of blood increases, our hearts have more work, and the heart muscle is stretched further. To avoid too much strain, the heart produces a hormone that triggers urine production in the kidneys. Therefore, the more we drink, the more urine we produce.

We lose about half a liter (one pint) of water through our lungs and skin. It may be hard to imagine how we lose water through our lungs, but if you breathe on a mirror, you can see how much moisture your exhaled breath contains. Now, multiply the small droplets stuck to the mirror by the eighteen thousand daily breaths we take, and you'll arrive at the half liter. The more we breathe, the more water we lose.

The way we lose a pint of water through our skin, on the other hand, is easy to imagine: humans sweat, even in the most mild of climates. We lose even more water through our skin when we sit sweating in the sauna, or when the temperature is in the extreme high digits. We can even lose liters of water on days we exercise heavily. And the elderly should be extra cautious on hot days, staying cool and in the shade when possible, since when we age, we tend to drink less fluid.

The fourth organ that eliminates water is the intestines. Even a perfectly formed bowel movement contains 6.5 to 10 ounces of water. If it's mushy or liquid, the stool can quickly reach a liter or more per day.

About half the water we need we receive through our food, and the other half we drink. If we don't supply our bodies with enough, they can make up for the lost water, at least temporarily. The body can shut down urine production, lower sweat production, and attempt to extract more water from the stool with a longer passage time. Reducing water loss through these organs is necessary to avoid collapsing altogether.

Proper digestion depends on the abundant production of digestive secretions. Saliva, gastric juices, bile, pancreatic fluid, and intestinal juices add up to eight to nine liters (nine to ten quarts) of liquid, which, fortunately, are absorbed in the body by the small intestine. Otherwise, we'd have to drink water continuously. When there's a lack of fluids, our bodies can reduce the production of these juices. You can see how this happens when your mouth is dry or you're constipated.

How does all this apply to the fitness program for the intestines? During the resting period, you won't get much water from the little food you eat, so you'll need to drink more! If you weigh 165 pounds, you have to drink at least 3 liters (3.2 quarts) of water per day. If you weigh 110 pounds, 2 liters (2.1 quarts) are enough, and if you're 220 pounds, then you'll need 4 liters (4.2 quarts) of water daily. This is 1 liter (1.1 quarts) for every 55 pounds. If you drink these amounts, you'll feel good during the resting part of the program. You have to also figure in the loss of water through sweat if you exercise or go to the sauna during this time.

You can tell if you've been drinking enough based on the color of your urine. If it's transparent with a touch of yellow, you're good to go. The darker the yellow, the more you need to drink!

BACK TO THE BOOKS—WE HAVE TO LEARN ABOUT GOOD DIGESTION

Chew Training Is Jogging for the Intestinally Enlightened

Good chewing is one of the most difficult tasks to learn if you didn't as a child. We don't entirely know why one person chews well and another swallows everything whole. We do know that eating behavior is learned at an early age. Children learn many behaviors by watching and copying the people around them. That means that if a child has parents who scarf down their food, it's highly likely that the child will do the same.

If only one of the parents eats too fast, then there's only a 50 percent chance that the child will too.

The number of siblings can also influence the child's eating behavior. If there are a lot of people gathered around the table, the child will feel the need to eat rapidly in order to get enough food and be full. During times when food is limited, people chew more to enjoy what little food is on the plate as much as possible. It's easy to assume the opposite situation these days, when food is available in excess.

The first important step is understanding how vital good chewing is for our intestines, and thus for our overall health. Think about the product that comes out below and what it says about our digestion.

However, just understanding this principle is not enough. We have to actually train with it in mind. If we don't practice something, then we can't actually do it, just like learning a language or a sport. Therefore, intensive chew training during your fitness program is the second important step.

The third step includes weekly chew training days for one to two years. If you quit training too soon, it only takes one to two months before you're swallowing your food whole again. It's just as if you crammed four weeks of vocabulary into your brain and then never practiced the language. After about two months, you'll have forgotten almost everything.

To avoid getting discouraged, imagine the favor you're doing for your intestines, liver, and overall health with good chewing. Think about how you're pulling the rug out from under all those nasty bacteria in your colon and how your skin and all your other organs will be overjoyed having to deal with fewer toxins as a result. It's going to help you!

Chew your way to health and beauty! And don't forget, it's about *good* chewing and not just *slow* chewing. Savor your food, and chew it until it's mushy; that's the important part.

We Have to Practice Feeling Full

The more tired your digestive tract is, the less it will relay the message of fullness. In Japan, one of the basic rules of eating healthily is to stop as soon as you feel a little full. But that's easier said than done, because often our stomachs can no longer transmit this information.

The only information that still arrives is, *We're stuffed; nothing else will fit!* In the case of a tired and sick stomach, we can fill it up to the top with food, like a sack. The feeling the stomach transmits is *bursting at the seams*. Being full should mean eating until the body is *satisfied*; there's a difference.

Where does the feeling of being full come from? After about twenty minutes, thorough chewing transmits a feeling of fullness, regardless of what and how much we ate. Fats and proteins also transmit this feeling. A baby's last sip of breast milk, which is full of fat, makes her full and happy. That's why babies who are bottle fed have trouble feeling full and satisfied from the beginning.

Carbohydrates don't make us feel full; they fill us up and make us fat. Low-fat snacks don't make us feel full; they just fill us up. If we strain our stomachs by eating too much, they get tired and can no longer tell us when we're full.

Additionally, when we're tired at night, our bodies no longer transmit a feeling of fullness. If you eat a five-course meal late in the evening, you'll be surprised that you can eat dessert and cheese as well. Try doing the same thing at lunch, when your stomach isn't getting ready for a night's rest. You'd feel full after the second course and want to go for a walk.

During your fitness program, you'll have the best opportunity to train yourself to recognize and feel a healthy feeling of fullness. It can take a couple of days before you notice it, but when you do, it's important to stop eating when you recognize it. The best part is you won't feel tired after eating anymore!

You Can Even Train Your Bowel Movement

Due to the effects of the Epsom salts you'll be drinking during the program, you won't be able to choose when you go to the bathroom. Not that the effect is explosive and you won't make it to the next toilet, but the need will be a little more intense, or at least clear enough to make you react quickly.

Things will look and feel a little different than normal. The mad rush in the morning often makes us ignore the need for a bowel movement. If this happens too often, the colon feels left out and also starts to ignore crucial signals on its end. When you're suffering from constipation, you should train your colon. To do this, go to the bathroom shortly after eating breakfast and show your bowel that the right moment has arrived. Even if it doesn't get it at first, and is possibly offended for a while, it'll be eternally grateful if you make a routine out of it.

Medical Assistance and the Role of the Stomach Treatment

The recommended training and rinsing helps a tired bowel. When it's time, however, to reactivate and regenerate tired sections of the intestines, or to treat diseases, resting and rinsing the digestive tract is often not enough.

In these cases, you should make use of a bowel specialist (gastroenterologist). The best option is to find one who is specially trained in the diagnostics and therapy based on the work of F. X. Mayr. There are about six hundred Mayr-trained therapists worldwide; with a little luck, one of them is nearby. You could also take a time-out and care for your intestines intensively in a specialized health center far away from daily life.

What can you expect from professional support? At first, the doctor or therapist needs to determine the condition of your digestive tract health. In the process, she'll see how much the bones in your chest and abdominal areas have changed already. She will also determine the epigastric angle that is built by the two sides of your rib cage. The two sides typically meet below the sternum at an angle of 20 to 40 degrees.

If the stomach under the left side of the rib cage is enlarged and the liver is jammed under the right side of the rib cage, they push the entire rib cage apart, since it's flexible and can adapt to its contents. The angle, in this case, can be 90 degrees or more.

Then the doctor will palpate (examine by touch) the size, location, and consistency of your small and large intestines and search for abnormal lymph accumulation in your abdominal area. She'll tap on your abdominal wall to look for irritations such as infections, oversensitive regions, and buildup of gas. She will then document existing posture modifications or damage. Based on the findings and possible intolerances, you will come up with a bland diet together that works for the upcoming program.

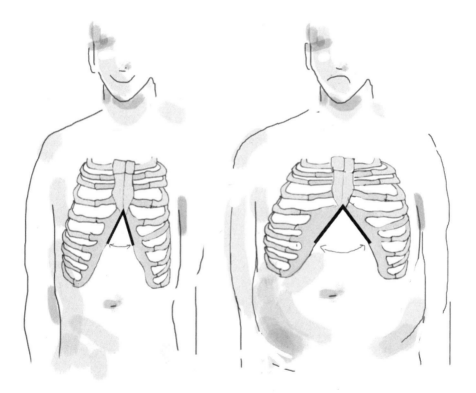

An integral part of this professionally accompanied intestinal fitness program is the manual stomach treatment, which consists of gently and rhythmically pressing the intestines for five to ten minutes.

Along with gurgling and grumbling noises, this triggers peristalsis, the absorption of nutrients, and the onward movement of gases. The manual stomach treatment also improves circulation and lymph drainage. The stomach grows surprisingly smaller in a short time. It regulates breathing, heart function, and blood pressure, and your skin's elasticity noticeably improves. This is how the intestines learn to function better. The worse the condition of your digestive tract is, the more important it is to carry out the treatment daily to stabilize its health.

FIT, FITTER, FITTEST—THE TEN-DAY FITNESS PROGRAM FOR YOUR INTESTINES AND OVERALL HEALTH

By now, you know that your eating behavior is key to a healthy bowel, and I know you're thinking, *No problem. I can chew exaggeratedly, stop snacking, and eat a small dinner, or occasionally no dinner at all. In a couple of months, my digestion will be fit as a fiddle.* But for many people, the fact that it takes months is a problem.

In this part, I am going to entrust you with a program that has stood the test of time. During the last twenty years working in this field, I've improved it through trial and error, and new experiences and studies have shaped the final product.

Whether the recommended ten days is enough for your intestines and overall health depends on several factors. The most important one is your current state of health, which determines whether or not you'll need professional support. If you've had any health issues, recently or for a while now, that affect your bowels or other organs, or you take medication on a regular basis, then you should ask a holistic bowel specialist to guide you through the program.

Another factor is what type of person you are when it comes to your health. Are you the kind of person who pushes their health to the limit, lives in excess, and expects to happily reach their ninetieth birthday anyway? Does that kind of person even exist? It's usually the people who live a life of moderation who reach a ripe old age. For people living in excess, it's often inconceivable to find the right balance. Unfortunately, this attitude doesn't change until a serious disease is looming on the horizon.

The good news is that most people are willing to change when they see the big picture. When they recognize how they deal with nutrition and health issues, they're already one step further in the right direction. So, how would you describe yourself? My personality types make use of Latin roots—*tox* represents toxins and *detox* represents detoxification. And *Lost* has nothing to do with the TV show.

The TOX type: He's as fearless as Tarzan and indulges himself in all kinds of bad eating habits. He thinks nothing can harm him. Like in the Stone Age, he only worries about basic survival; he likes to claim they didn't have healthy options back then either. The problem is, he seems to forget that, back then, they didn't have overabundant amounts of sugar or a fast food restaurant on every corner. He also believes in quack doctors who supposedly know how to handle the consequences of his lifestyle. If he survives his first heart attack, there's a chance he'll start caring about what he eats and how he treats his intestines. He might become a new man. An intestinal fitness program for TOX types is out of the question. Maybe he suffers from his delusional vitality that has long kept him alive, or from the fact that his body tells him too late when it's had enough.

The TOX-DETOX type: She likes doing the wrong thing and is quite aware of the possible consequences. She loves her lifestyle, but realizes that, health-wise, she can't go on like this forever. She might have already noticed that her body needs a break. With every detox program she tries, she promises herself she'll change, but in the end, her lack of willpower prevails. Anyway, she doesn't notice any improvements. But if the breaks are long enough, and she manages to complete a program now and then, keeping the toxification and detoxification in balance, the TOX-DETOX type will be able to lead a long life. For this type of person, the intestinal fitness program becomes a life-long companion.

The DETOX type: He is the definition of a healthy person. He enjoys eating in moderation, knows a lot about nutrition, and exercises regularly. Health-wise, nothing surprises him. If he makes a mistake, he immediately fixes it with the appropriate information. He takes breaks, because he notices when his battery is only 80 percent charged. During the intestinal fitness program, he learns what nutrition has to do with his bowel and then applies it to his daily life. The program solidifies his already-remarkable health consciousness. He's happy to do it in order to become even fitter.

The LOST type: She's endlessly searching for new diets to either lose weight or permanently keep health problems under control. She never finds a healthy foundation. Her attempts are usually extreme and not sustainably viable. The LOST type is always open to new programs. My program could help stabilize her health and weight.

You may be a combination of some of these personality types. Keep in mind, this is by no means an exhaustive list.

THE TEN-DAY INTESTINAL DETOX PROGRAM

Some people claim the largest problem with doing this kind of detox program daily at home is a full refrigerator. In a single person's home, it's easy to empty the fridge. When the rest of the family would like to keep eating, however, it's a little more difficult to commit to the program and resist temptation.

And that's exactly the problem—if you don't feel like watching everyone eat while you're fasting (or eating less), you'll be isolated from friends, family, and others. Members of religious communities have it easier, because they have special times for fasting together.

There's an easy solution: find a few accomplices! Ask friends or family to join in and set a start date. Meet up regularly during the program and exchange stories. That'll make it easier to keep going and share your successes.

What if you're surrounded by a bunch of TOX types? Well, maybe you can convince them to take the plunge. They'll thank you for it later, once they experience the positive effect the program has on their bodies.

What You Need and What You Don't

First of all, you'll need ten stress-free days and the prospect of sleeping eight hours every night. There's no room for overly exhausting phases at work or home! As mentioned before, it's a real added bonus if as many friends or family members participate as possible. And you're going to need thirty minutes, two times a day, for your meals, so the chew training works.

What else do you need? You'll need enough water (with as little carbonation as possible) and some herbal teas that you like. There's an endless list of delicious options, such as lemongrass, Greek mountain tea, alkaline teas (like chamomile), detox teas, and more.

For your meals, you're always going to need a "chew trainer" and nutritious and vitamin-rich food. I call this kind of food "Go's," and the food you should avoid, "No-Go's." Choose what looks good to you, but try not to switch too often. Monotonous food is gentler on your stomach than a varied diet.

Foods that are suitable for chew training are all kinds of nuts, coconut, dry spelt bread, or gluten-free bread. If you choose the bread, you should slice it when it's fresh and then let it dry two to three days, until it's hard and stale.

Go's are almond milk; soy milk; raw milk; yogurt made from the milk of sheep, goats, or cows (or coconut or soy); homemade green smoothies; and root vegetable juice.

If you cannot follow a strict diet due to a medical condition, or you do not want to lose weight under any circumstances, additional Go's you can eat are avocados, turkey breast, wild salmon, soft-boiled eggs, vegetable soup, and vegetables that are easily digested and don't cause bloating.

There are four No-Go's that are absolutely taboo while you're detoxing, cleansing, and resting your intestines—cigarettes, coffee, alcohol, and sugar. If you're a TOX type, this must sound horrible to you! But be brave—dare to change.

Everyone is familiar with the health risks of smoking. Nicotine also has a stimulating effect on the bowel, which some smokers with tired intestines use to trigger a bowel movement. These irritants are counterproductive during the resting phase, which is one of many reasons you'll need to do without.

As a smoker, if you train your eating habits for ten days or longer, you won't gain weight, even if you quit smoking afterward. I promise! There's no better time to quit. It's worth thinking about!

From a medical perspective, there are no arguments against a moderate consumption of coffee. But it also irritates the intestines and is therefore taboo during the program. It stimulates the sympathetic nervous system, like alcohol and cigarettes, and during regeneration, it's the parasympathetic nervous system we need. Furthermore, we need to sleep soundly during this period, so it's best to do without coffee.

For many people, coffee withdrawal leads to a headache in the first three days, so it's better to quit drinking it a week before you begin the program. You'll still get a headache, but much less than if you quit while changing your eating habits.

Small amounts of alcohol per day are normally acceptable, but you need to do without during the program. Your liver will be happy about the break from alcohol detoxification. Besides, the consumption of alcohol reduces the histamine-neutralizing enzyme amine oxidase. Even if you don't consume any histamines during the program, it appears that alcohol influences digestion, and you don't want that during the resting period.

Sugar is poison! The damage sugar causes is as wide-ranging as the damage alcohol and cigarettes cause. Of course, it also depends on quantity. During your fitness program, it would attack your metabolism and lead to hypoglycemia (deficiency of glucose in the bloodstream), which transmits feelings of hunger and a desire to eat. Sugar is a chemical product that disrupts our metabolism. This leads to a vitamin B deficiency and digestive disorders. In very limited amounts, it's fine in your everyday life, but it has no business in your detox program.

Kick It First!

A week before starting the program, you'll need to slowly get prepared. If you have to continue to work during the program, this preliminary week is especially important. It keeps you from feeling bad the first few days. During this preparatory week, if possible, start your day with three grams of Epsom salts (one level teaspoon) in one-quarter of a liter (about eight fluid ounces) of warm water on an empty stomach.

Then, chew your usual breakfast and lunch exaggeratedly well and reduce the size of your dinner significantly. If you can, quit eating dinner altogether. While doing this, you absorb less water from your food, so it's important to drink two to three liters of unsweetened tea or water every day. Additionally, leave coffee alone, and reduce your intake of alcohol and cigarettes, or quit entirely if possible.

During this week of preparation, drink one-quarter of a liter (about eight fluid ounces) of water mixed with a slightly heaped teaspoon of alkaline powder two times daily. This will help ease the withdrawal process and ensure that you'll feel fine during the next ten days.

The Ten Days

Ideally, you should start the program on a Friday. You can handle the first day easily, even if you're working. The second and third days are a little trickier, but it'll be the weekend, so choose a quiet one. From the fourth to the tenth day, everything will run like clockwork, because your body will have understood that something has changed, and you'll feel better with each new day.

Rinsing: Get rid of that crap! You're going to see what a great feeling it is when the intestines are flushed out entirely. Every day begins with an Epsom salt rinse, three grams (one level teaspoon) in one-quarter of a liter (about eight fluid ounces) of water, right after you get up. You'll see how your bowel reacts in the first three days, or you already witnessed it during the preparation week. One to three times a day, you should have a mushy to liquid bowel movement, and the stench decreases every day more and more. If you suffer from constipation, take a double dose for the first two days.

If you're not satisfied with the results of rinsing, you can drink another portion of Epsom salts a half hour before lunch.

Breakfast and lunch: You need to plan on thirty minutes for your meals. A healthy feeling of fullness usually kicks in after about twenty minutes, but it can take longer in the beginning. This feeling doesn't last long if you eat in a hurry and chew poorly, not to mention it's not as gentle on your bowel and makes the program unnecessarily difficult.

Don't forget, your goal is to give the intestinal germs nothing to eat. And you shouldn't only chew well; you should chew exaggeratedly well! The meals always consist of a chew trainer and a food from the Go list that provides you with additional vitamins, minerals, and trace elements, or a few extra calories if you want to avoid losing weight. The Go's need the saliva produced from the chew trainer to be digested easily, because they're also hard to chew. The less fiber the food contains, the better.

What happens during a meal? You put the chew trainer, a nut or a bit of air-dried bread, into your mouth and chew until only a saliva mush is left. Then add a small amount of the

Go-list food to the mush in your mouth and continue chewing until the bite disappears. Keep doing this bite by bite until you feel slightly full. Don't drink anything while eating, because it reduces the resting effect.

Eat the same food for lunch that you did for breakfast. The more monotonous it is, the gentler it is. If you decide to go with the milder version of this program (for medical reasons or worries about weight loss) and eat vegetable soup or vegetables for lunch, you should keep it as monotonous as possible. For example, don't eat more than two kinds of vegetables, such as potatoes and carrots or potatoes and fennel. Avoid eating coarse-fibered vegetables that make you feel bloated, like leeks, cabbage, kale, onions, and legumes.

Whatever you do, don't prepare a colorful veggie plate for lunch, because the more varied the diet, the higher the risk that something is in there that you won't tolerate well, thereby canceling out the resting effect. Add a chew trainer to the vegetables you select, because you won't feel full for long otherwise.

Between meals: Drink two to three liters (about sixty-five to one hundred ounces) between meals every day and begin doing so about half an hour after a meal. If you sweat a lot (from exercise, sauna, etc.), make sure to add the lost fluids to the equation. A person with normally functioning skin loses about half a liter (one pint) of sweat per sauna visit. A little exercise and two times in a sauna, and you've already lost 3.5 to 4.5 liters (4 to 5 quarts) of fluids. Your well-being depends on drinking enough liquids—even more now than it does in daily life. The kidneys are an excellent detox organ, so make them work!

And your stomach? If you're lucky enough to live close to a holistic intestinal specialist, and you decided to have professional help during the program, you'll receive three to five medical stomach treatments based on the work of Mayr. This also means that, after talking to your doctor, you can switch to a longer program if you're having more trouble with digestion or your overall health. Since the program is usually only difficult in the beginning, if you need to extend, it should be easy as pie to accomplish.

Athletics, wellness, and sauna: Exercise a little less during the program than you normally would. If you don't exercise anyway, right now, you're probably thinking, *Perfect!* But don't misunderstand; if you're a lazybones, you need to change. Now is the time to add a little more movement to your life. There are easy options beyond going to a gym. You can take the stairs instead of the elevator, and you can walk to your destination if it isn't too far away. If it's just around the corner or one bus stop away, get out there and pound the pavement.

During the program, you'll have plenty of motivation and energy. The one thing, though, that often disappears with less food is your endurance. That's why you need to alternate days of exercise and rest. Your goal is regeneration and detoxification, so preparing for your next marathon can wait ten days.

Sauna visits or steam baths can aid in detoxifying your skin. Doing this expels the nicotine from your body in overdrive, taking away your desire to smoke (hopefully). For the first couple of days, your sweat is often sticky and smells bad, but that disappears soon.

Hangry in the evening: Skipping dinner is difficult during these ten days. But once you make it past the first phase, you can succeed in skipping dinner permanently. I have many patients who have always had weight problems—aggravated by a slow metabolic rate—and get it under control by skipping dinner. Interestingly enough, this doesn't work when you skip breakfast. To get your metabolic rate, we label and measure the daily amounts of energy that your body needs to keep everything functioning well. If you have a slow metabolic rate, you need fewer calories, and if you're not careful about what you eat, you can gain weight rather quickly.

It's hard to break a habit, and eating (or rather overeating) is one of the most difficult habits to break. For this reason, the little "habit hobbit" in your stomach is going to interject and demand what he thinks he needs: *What the heck are you doing? It would be so much more enjoyable if you ate something delicious, drank a nice glass of red wine, and wrapped it all up with a soothing cigarette! After all, you only live once! How stupid can you be?!*

But at the moment, you're not only concerned about enjoying yourself; you decided to partake in this program to stay or become healthy. With your goal in plain view, answer the hobbit with, "No thanks, but if you're quiet now, you might get what you want again soon." Then raise a glass of water or tea to his health. Your little habit hobbit will quickly figure out what you're doing, and in two or three days, he'll leave you alone. Some habit hobbits are a little slow catching on, but they will eventually get it and respect your decision. If you're a repeat offender—you've done this before—then you'll know that the hobbit usually pipes down soon enough.

A fundamental principle of this ten-day detox program is to leave your intestines alone in the evening! Herbal tea, water, or a tasty vegetable broth are allowed and will help you suppress your hunger. On top of that, you can spoon-feed yourself the tea or broth to transmit the feeling of eating something. This way, it should be easier to avoid withdrawal symptoms.

The Aftermath

The ten days are over, and it was easier than you thought. You've learned to eat in moderation and quit once you feel slightly full. You also stopped snacking, left your intestines alone in the evenings, and drank ample fluids. You dropped the No-Go's, and you feel invigorated and cleansed. When you wake up in the morning, you're wide awake and ready to go—the way it should be after a good night's rest.

Depending on what type of person you are, you may have even decided to change your eating behavior for good. But be careful and take it one step at a time, because it's possible to change a lot in a short time, but you'll soon notice that you're overwhelmed with it all. And then you might slip back into your old habits. Therefore, you should change one thing at a time and concentrate on maintaining that good habit for a while before making the next change.

If you're not one of the few people who have always chewed well, learning to master the thorough chew technique is the most difficult task in my opinion, but also the most rewarding for your health. If you can set aside one day a week to concentrate on your chewing during a normal lunch and then skip dinner, it will help you a great deal.

During the week after your program, continue the chew training every day by exaggeratedly chewing nuts and old bread. You'll be back to eating regular meals again, which you should also continue to exaggeratedly chew. This step is training for the advanced level, which you've already achieved!

Start adding easily digestible fruit to your breakfast. Bananas, papaya, blueberries, or a little mango are especially suitable. Eggs are also allowed again.

For lunch, try to eat easily digestible, non-bloating vegetables and, as a side, some fish, poultry, rice, or pasta. Three-quarters of the plate should always be reserved for vegetables, and the other quarter can be whatever mix of sides you want.

You should try to skip dinner for a few more days after finishing the program, phasing it back in slowly rather than burdening your intestines with a sudden change in their work schedule. And when you do start eating dinner again, stick to vegetable soup at first.

During this first week after the program, be sure to continue drinking Epsom salts before breakfast, but every other day now. Also keep drinking the alkaline powder mixture twice a day, mornings and midday, thirty minutes before you eat.

Training—And a Day of Rest for Your Intestines

In the wonderful BBC documentary *Eat, Fast and Live Longer,* reporter Michael Mosley was looking for a way to be done with all lifestyle diseases caused by overindulging in food, such as heart attacks, strokes, diabetes, and cancer.

When I first heard of this documentary, I thought I had been on the wrong path for twenty years. Can we really eat fast and live longer at the same time? But then I looked more closely at the title and breathed a sigh of relief, realizing just how important commas can be.

Mosley is convinced of the positive effects of fasting but cannot fathom changing his lifestyle. Therefore, he suggests leading your life as usual for five days of the week and fasting for the other two days (no food at all). It's hard to imagine how that can help people in the long run. The first day of fasting is unpleasant, but by the second day it is just plain excruciating. Your body goes through ultimate fatigue. It's hard to think, your limbs are tired, and headaches are frequent. If you had to put up with this fifty-two times a year, you'd be saying, "I prefer to die earlier!"

If this doesn't sound like something you'd like to sign up for, I'd recommend the practice of one day of "resting" each week, which has proven to work quite well. You chew your normal breakfast and lunch exaggeratedly, which means you eat a lot less and still feel full, and you skip dinner. Not having any food after lunch means you leave your bowels to "rest" until the next morning. This method of fasting also calls for chew training, which will help you chew correctly, automatically, and remain stomach- and bowel-friendly forever. It's important to choose a day and stick to it. The same day should always be marked on your calendar. Don't let fate decide, because there are a million reasons to keep postponing what you know should be done.

For many people, Monday is the best "resting day" to recuperate from the weekend. But Sunday is also a good choice, because you can eat breakfast and lunch a little later. Then it's not so hard to skip eating solid foods in the evening. In the morning on the day you choose, a small dose of Epsom salts on an empty stomach has been proven to help improve intestinal peristalsis, and it also rinses the bowel a bit.

And My Weight?

The primary goals of the ten-day fitness program are the regeneration of your intestines and detoxification. During this time, you will eat less than five hundred calories on a daily basis and, as a result, lose weight. Luckily, you won't go hungry, because you'll be chewing very well. Depending on your metabolic rate and additional burned energy from exercise, that adds up to about three to nine pounds of fat in ten days.

As long as you have fat reserves, your body generates vital energy from these reserves when you're not eating. When these fat reserves are depleted, your body grabs energy from protein, thereby deteriorating the muscles as well as other parts of the body. Obviously, you shouldn't let it come to this. During these ten days, if you exercise less than usual, you'll lose muscle, and if you work out more, you'll build muscle. It's the same principle as when you're eating a normal diet.

The diet during these ten days is relatively low sodium, which means, in the first few days, you'll lose water that was stored in your tissues. Salt absorbs water in the body; it holds on to it. If you usually like to eat salty meals, you can add up to four liters (about a gallon) of water loss to the fat loss. That means, weight loss during the program can be from three to eighteen pounds, but some of that will be water weight.

If you were to go back to eating just as much salt immediately after the ten days, you would gain back the water in your tissues. And if you went back to your old eating habits, within a few weeks you'd gain back the weight you lost during the program.

Your body weight precisely reflects, when, what, and how much you eat and how much you exercise. Yet many people still try one diet after the other without changing anything permanently and then wonder why they can't lose weight (or even gain it). With all that we know about weight gain and diet, you'd think most people would know that this yo-yo dieting is useless for weight loss if they don't fundamentally change something in their eating habits. During a low-calorie diet, the body switches on the *Help, I'm starving!* button, and your metabolism shuts down. Once the diet ends, if you immediately start eating the same way you did before, your body stores everything it can at first, just in case you switch the button back on.

Getting back to our program, weigh yourself at the beginning and the end of the ten days. Make sure your stomach is empty and you've emptied your bowels and your bladder. Weighing yourself daily makes no sense and will drive you crazy. Since you're drinking a lot, your weight will fluctuate with all those fluids. So you're eating very little and weigh a few pounds more? No wonder, because the water you drank hasn't left your body through your bladder yet. Daily weight checks are not exactly motivating.

Here's a scenario from everyday life. You had a special event last night. You ate well and in excess. They didn't exactly hold back on the salt, since it makes food tastier and makes you want to drink more. The salt shoots water into your tissues, and that's where you find it the next morning when you go to weigh yourself after a bowel movement and . . . what's this?! You weigh four pounds more than you did twenty-four hours ago. The day can't get any worse. But the four pounds are mostly "just" water. Two pounds of fat is equal to approximately eight thousand calories. If your weight gain had been fat, you'd have eaten sixteen thousand calories too much. That would be about eleven pounds of steak and seventeen pounds of potatoes and carrots. It's hard to believe anyone could eat that much!

Permanent weight loss depends on what you eat, how you eat, and when you eat. The following have significant influence:

sugar (this does not refer to the piece of chocolate you eat after lunch)
wheat, especially bread and pasta
snacking
dinner as your main meal
chewing

Therefore, avoid beverage-industry drinks (full of sugar!), eat little bread and other wheat products, chew well (you eat less and feel full longer), try not to snack between meals, and eat as little as possible for dinner. If you follow these guidelines, you'll reach the right weight for your body, without exception.

All the beauty magazines talk endlessly about working out and how exercise is good for your muscles and circulation. And they're right, but it won't help you lose weight permanently. If you don't change your eating habits at the same time, your weight won't stabilize.

That piece of cake you've been eyeing is not going to help you lose weight just because you had a great workout. If you exercised a ton, you could lose weight temporarily. But since you probably won't be working out that intensely every week for the next couple of decades, an athletic fitness program won't help you keep the weight off forever.

If you don't change your eating habits, the number on the scale will slowly creep up again. If it does, you'll be understandably frustrated and want to eat another piece of cake. The vicious circle has been perfectly formed, and you're in a bad mood and hungry.

ADVICE AND RECIPES SUMMED UP

Stuff to Consider

Here's a list of preliminary medical tests you should consider before you start my detox program, especially if you have any health issues:

- breath test to check for fructose and lactose intolerance
- measure the level of histamines and amine oxidase in the blood
- test for celiac disease
- signs of zonulin in blood or stool
- signs of blood and tumor M2 pyruvate kinase in stool
- ultrasound of the abdominal area
- colonoscopy

If anything comes up positive, make sure you only do the program with the support of a doctor!

And here is a list of No-Go's during the program:

- cigarettes
- alcohol
- coffee
- sugar

During the preparation week:

- quit the No-Go's
- start your chew training, so you can begin to eat less but will still feel full sooner
- drink Epsom salts every morning (one level teaspoon dissolved in warm water)
- take alkaline powder morning and midday (one slightly heaped teaspoon dissolved in water)
- no dinner, or significantly less

This week is to help you get used to what awaits you during the program, so it's not as difficult when you start. Here's what you will need during the ten-day program:

- understanding friends
- thirty minutes for every meal
- Epsom salts
- alkaline powder
- chew trainers, so you're full sooner and your stomach doesn't have to work so hard
  - large chunks of coconut chips
  - almonds
  - walnuts
  - dry spelt bread or dry gluten-free bread

- Go's
  - almond or other nut milk
  - yogurt (made from soy or sheep's, cow's, or coconut milk)
  - raw milk
  - homemade red or green smoothies (see the recipes on the next page)
  - root vegetable juice or root vegetable broth

What else is good for you during this week (or the week after):

- bananas, papayas, blueberries, avocados
- oatmeal or millet porridge
- non-bloating vegetables
- rice
- fish or poultry

Here are grocery shopping tips before you start the week:

- unsalted(!) nuts and organic vegetables
- bread should be made of spelt (under no circumstances whole-grain products)
- always raw milk
- alkaline powder
- Epsom salts

Easy Recipes to Try During Detox Week

Homemade nut milk
Nut milk will keep 4 to 5 days in the refrigerator.
Makes 3 cups.

1 cup blanched almonds or walnuts
1 large or 2 small dates, pitted
1½ cups water

1½ cups coconut water
Cheesecloth or sieve

Soak the nuts in a bowl of water overnight, making sure the water covers the nuts. Drain the water, reserving 1½ cups if possible (supplement with fresh water if necessary). Place the nuts and dates in a blender or food processor, along with a bit of the nut water, and blend for about 30 seconds. Add the remaining water, along with the coconut water, and blend until you achieve a smooth consistency. Filter the nut milk through cheesecloth or a fine sieve. Stir before drinking.

Red smoothie (breakfast)

Here's a super easy drink to make in the mornings that also packs a powerful punch of antioxidants from the berries and coconut water.
Approximately 100 calories, 3 grams fructose

½ average-sized organic banana
1 handful of organic blueberries
½ teaspoon almond butter
¾ cup coconut water

Throw all the ingredients in a blender and you're good to go!

Green smoothie (lunch)

Approximately 250 calories.

1 cup arugula or mixed wild herbs (dandelion, daisy, clover, stinging nettle, or whatever is growing at the moment are great options for herbs)
1 cup spinach or beet leaves
½ avocado
½ banana

¾ cup coconut water (less if a thicker consistency is desired)
a pinch of salt and pepper

Throw it all in the blender and you're good to go!

Vegetable broth

8½ cups water (about 2 quarts)
about 1½ pounds fresh vegetable roots (celery root, parsley root, carrots, fennel, parsnips)
1 bunch of parsley
1 teaspoon peppercorns
1 cup mixed herbs (dandelion, daisy, clover, stinging nettle, or whatever is available and growing at the moment)

In a large pot, bring the water to a gentle boil. Finely chop all ingredients and add them to the pot of hot water. Lower temp and simmer for around 30 minutes. Strain through a sieve to collect just the hot broth. Season with salt and pepper and any other organic seasoning you desire (no MSG).

EAT WHAT YOU CAN DIGEST—THE RIGHT DIET FOR YOU AND YOUR INTESTINES

Nutritious, natural food is an important prerequisite for being healthy, getting healthy, and remaining healthy. It is an essential foundation for the body to be able to heal itself.

Hardly any other topic in medicine is as debated as healthy food—probably because there are many ways to eat healthily. Humans are capable of adapting and have shown over thousands of years that they can survive under even the most extreme conditions. But there are a few prerequisites that they have to fulfill first.

Access to high-quality food has to be guaranteed. The food has to be digestible, and we must eat in moderation. Overindulgence is the source of many diseases. When asked what the secret to a long, healthy life is,

Jiroemon Kimura replied, "Eating in moderation." The Japanese man died at the age of nearly 117. Excessive eating and poor digestion go hand in hand; we can smell it on the toilet and see it in our stool.

Above all, we have to beware of making a fatal mistake: it's not enough to feed our bodies healthy food—our intestines also have to break this food down into the smallest components possible and supply our bodies with these nutrients. That means if our digestion isn't working properly, we're not eating healthily no matter what we're ingesting. If the digestive tract is tired and underperforming, it needs to complete a fitness program to strengthen itself. Otherwise, it might not be able to convert even the highest quality of food into useful energy.

What options do we have when selecting produce that's right for us? To answer this question, it's essential to remember what nourishment patterns humans have adopted over the last few thousand years. This will start us off in the right direction.

Imagine fish in an aquarium. They are used to a specific diet. If you feed them something you find randomly in your kitchen, you'll probably find most of them floating on the surface the next day.

Now, we're clearly not fish; we can eat a lot more than fish can. But our food and eating behavior has changed more in the last fifty years than during the thousands of years before. When we consider the number of modern people with metabolic diseases such as gout and diabetes, cardiovascular diseases that begin with high blood pressure and end in strokes or heart attacks, and diet-related cancerous diseases, we have to admit that we're doing something wrong.

What exactly has changed so drastically in our diets? The numbers can give us a clue: We eat *twice as much* meat and sugar than people did one hundred years ago; we consume mountains of dairy products that were only available in small amounts just 150 years ago. Furthermore, food industry processes have changed a large part of our food to such an extent that our intestines don't know what to do with it; they can't recognize any patterns.

On top of that, our bowels receive too much and too often. We've forgotten the natural rhythm of our intestines. We eat too fast, too often, and at the wrong times. In every culture, the correct times to eat have been passed on through sayings: Eat breakfast like a king, lunch like a prince, and dinner like a pauper. The Spaniards phrase it more drastically: *De grandes cenas están las tumbas llenas*, meaning *large dinners fill the coffins*.

We liken people's diets in the Mediterranean region with the Mediterranean diet, which, after much research, is considered one of the healthiest diets around. But we shouldn't forget that these countries haven't really been following a Mediterranean diet for about sixty years now. When looking at statistics on cases of cardiovascular and tumor diseases, it looks just as bad in these countries now as it does in America. Heavy dinners are only a part of the problem.

We have to rediscover the right rhythm! On top of that, we need to eat the right produce in the right amounts.

Our selection always has to focus on the performance of our digestive organs. No one can tell you with absolute certainty what your diet should look like, because everyone's digestive tract is different. There are preferences and habits that always have to be taken into consideration.

That's why you might be sick of diets. Diets are usually suggested for everyone, and that's not possible.

There are two kinds of recommended diets. One of them is about losing weight and nothing else. These diets are usually done for a limited time, and if everything goes back to normal when we're "finished" losing weight, nothing changes in the end because the weight comes back after we go off the diet. If you were to eat according to these diets your entire life, you'd get sick of them soon, not to mention that they're sometimes really unhealthy. Nutritious, easily digestible food is something else; it's a lifelong diet.

The other kind of diet consists of very extreme, one-sided recommendations and isn't for everyone. One example is Max Otto Bruker's whole-foods diet, rich in vital substances. He was a German doctor who propagated food that has been processed or refined as little as possible. In general, this is a good idea. However, the coarse whole-grain products have clogged a tired, underperforming bowel or two. Really tired intestines profited for a while, because gas-producing bacterial processes caused by the whole grains shortened the digestion time. But whipping a tired donkey through the prairie doesn't work for very long.

My recommendation? You can eat whatever agrees with you as long as you chew well, so you can digest well, and eat in moderation! Don't snack between meals, and when you're tired, eat as little as possible. Your daily nutrition should be fundamentally healthy, but that doesn't mean you can't happily make an exception once in a while—we're all human. Just remember that the exceptions shouldn't become the rule.

I'd like to focus on various foods now and inform you about their nutritional value, digestibility, and the correct amount to consume.

Alcohol

In many cultures, alcoholic drinks are a part of daily meals. Humans discovered the intoxicating effects of fermented fruit and wheat many thousands of years ago. Right after coffee and water, alcoholic drinks are number three on our list of most-consumed drinks.

The health risks from drinking alcohol are generally played down. Most people are unfamiliar with the impact it has on our digestive tract. We know it can be addictive, but that hasn't changed the way we handle it. According to some estimates, there are almost thirty-two million Americans who have had a serious drinking problem in the last year alone.

Even if drinking very small amounts of alcohol every day supposedly lowers the risk of having a heart attack, large amounts have the opposite effect and are frequently the cause for cardiac arrhythmias. Barely anyone knows that larger amounts of alcohol raise your risk of developing one of the many malignant diseases of the digestive tract. Also, cancer of the mouth, throat, larynx, and esophagus are just as common as cancer of the liver and colon—all places the alcohol travels through as we consume it.

Alcohol does not cause cancer directly, but it makes the cells weaker against cancer-causing substances. It irritates the mucous membrane, and its metabolic byproducts are toxic.

The stomach and small intestine absorb alcohol and start breaking it down, just as it is broken down later in the liver, with an enzyme, alcohol dehydrogenase. This is how alcohol transforms into the more toxic acetaldehyde.

A lot of the organ damage caused by chronic alcohol abuse can be traced back to a damaged small intestine mucosa. This mucous membrane becomes more permeable to partially broken-down nutrients that trigger an immune response from the body. A damaged small intestine facilitates the growth of bacteria that normally wouldn't be there. A chronically inflamed pancreas and cirrhosis of the liver (thirty-one thousand people die of this every year in America) are common results of alcohol abuse.

We cannot foresee who will become addicted and who will be spared; it depends on many factors. Environment, behavioral norms, and individual tolerance are important factors that determine one's path. For some, one glass of red wine can be just as bad as a bottle of red wine is for others. That is why it is medically unjustifiable to describe any amount as "harmless," let alone "healthy" for everyone. Hence, it's also impossible to specify the right amount in general.

If you're having any trouble at all with your digestive tract while drinking alcohol regularly, it would be wise to quit drinking it for a while and see if your issues improve or clear up entirely.

Fiber

Fiber resists digestion and is a wonderful thing. It accumulates in the large intestine, triggers intestinal peristalsis, makes digestion time shorter, and, therefore, lowers the chance that bad bacteria produce bad toxins. Additionally, fiber is able to absorb any toxins that do get produced, which lowers the risk of developing colon cancer.

Fruits and vegetables are fiber-rich foods. And it's important that the fruits and vegetables on your plate are as fresh as possible, because the vitamins, minerals, and trace elements they contain are just as important. These vital substances decrease when the fruits or vegetables sit in shipping containers for a long time or are left at room temperature too long. That's why it's best to buy as locally as possible. If there's not enough selection of local produce, eat frozen organic vegetables as your backup.

Except for legumes, there are no limitations as to the amount of vegetables you can eat. You can stop when you feel full. With fruit, it's another story. Fruit has always been a side dish for humans. It contains relatively high levels of fructose, which can only be absorbed in limited amounts and affects the body negatively. Fruit is healthy, but only in small quantities. You can easily figure out the right amount for yourself. Did you pass a lot of gas? If yes, then it was too much. Even a little bit of fruit can crank up the gas production in the evening, so it's better to eat it in the morning.

Bread

The bestsellers *Wheat Belly* by William Davis and *Grain Brain* by David Perlmutter and Kristin Loberg taught us to be afraid of bread. Today, when you're standing in a bakery, you'll see some passersby turning their heads away, like vegans in front of a butcher shop.

Bread is now practically classified as poison, but in America, bread consumption has increased by 29 percent in the past fifty years. In the Middle Ages, we ate five times more bread than we do today. So it can't be the quantity of bread that has something to do with our lifestyle diseases, but rather the quality. As previously presented, wheat really is problematic, but these days we have enough bread made of other grains to choose from.

There is, however, one reason to completely quit eating bread— celiac disease, the inflammation of the intestinal mucosa due to wheat intolerance. Even if you don't have celiac disease, gluten may still cause trouble if your intestines are already damaged. Plus, if you start having any medical issues with your digestion, skin, or immune system, temporarily going without bread will help you see if the conditions are related.

Depending on the person, there may be one more reason to not eat more than a slice of bread each day: if you want to lose weight, you aren't doing it by indulging in bread since it has a relatively high caloric value. Bread contains a lot of carbohydrates, which stimulate insulin secretions, and insulin affects your metabolism and your weight.

It wouldn't be realistic (not to mention any fun) to quit eating bread permanently, because we humans enjoy eating it. So why not get used to the right amount from the beginning?

If you have perfect digestion, without constant flatulence, and like to eat whole-grain spelt bread, then keep eating it. But if your digestion is already a little tired, like most people's in the Western world, grab some white spelt bread instead.

And don't worry if you want to skip it altogether; we don't really need bread to stay healthy. On the contrary, it's problematic when trying to maintain or lose weight, and too much gluten can even harm our health. Bread wasn't on the menu until about ten thousand years ago, which is pretty recent in the grand scheme of things. So it can't hurt to eat less bread.

Proteins

Proteins are the most important component for muscle mass and endless other substances, such as hormones and enzymes that control our metabolism.

Plants contain abundant amounts of protein. Seaweed is made of 65 percent protein! Legumes, nuts, and soy products all contain as much protein as meat, fish, or eggs. Spelt, oats, millet, and quinoa contain protein, and even vegetables are made of 5 to 10 percent protein. The right quantity is determined by your feeling of fullness. There is no research that has been able to justify restraint when eating vegetable proteins.

It's another story when it comes to animal proteins. Animal experiments have shown that large amounts of casein, the protein found in dairy products, stimulates the growth of tumors. We consume at least ten times more dairy products than we did one hundred years ago. Large amounts of animal protein have become the main part of many people's diets, and we know that animal protein increases IGF-1 (insulin-like growth factor), and with it, the risk of developing cancer or cardiovascular disease.

The problem is not the meat or the cheese—it's the quantity. Eating meat, fish, or cheese once or twice a week is enough. You can replace milk with almond milk (or another nut), and yogurt with soy or coconut yogurt. If you eat meat or fish at lunch, you should avoid eating cheese, cold cuts, yogurt, or milk the same day.

Fats

Don't be afraid of fats and oils! Like proteins, there are animal and vegetable fats, and the latter should always be given preference. Fat delivers energy, insulates against the cold, releases vitamins, protects inner organs as well as the nervous system (basically every cell), and pleases our taste buds.

"But it makes you gain weight," you might argue. No, fats don't make you gain weight! For decades, we've heard that fats and oils make us heavy and sick. Cardiovascular diseases, tumors, and pretty much all lifestyle diseases were supposedly caused by consuming fats. There has not been one study that supports this claim. Fats make you full, which is why we can't and don't want to eat really large amounts of them.

Thanks to the weight-loss craze, we were told to reduce our intake of fats and increase carbohydrates. The result was that many people became obese. Fats trigger a high flow of bile, which digests the fats and prevents gallstones from forming as easily.

Fats are made of various fatty acids. Our bodies can produce some of these fatty acids on their own, and others they cannot; these we need to absorb through the food we eat. That is why we call these fatty acids "essential fatty acids." Among other things, they are an important component of the cell membrane, are necessary to maintain vital brain functions, and improve the immune response.

In the group of polyunsaturated fatty acids, omega-3 fatty acids are especially valuable essential fatty acids. They're pure nutrition for the nerves! You can find these fatty acids especially in cold-pressed, unadulterated linseed oil, walnut and other nut oils, mustard seed oil, and canola oil. Since linseed has the best composition of fatty acids, you should eat two teaspoons of it every day. But you shouldn't just drink it; if you do, it will shut down your stomach and hamper digestion of the food that follows. You can pour it over your breakfast cereal or vegetables; it tastes delicious. Make sure not to heat up any of the above mentioned oils.

A note on oil in general: Cooking with olive oil is an integral part of the Mediterranean diet. It might not contain much of the omega-3 fatty acids, but it is just as healthy and works well for cooking (except when searing, because it can't get too hot). Be sure to add good-quality olive oil to your cooking routine.

Fish

Fish has always been on the human menu. In particular, it prevents artery calcification. People who eat fish regularly have fewer heart attacks and strokes. According to the latest information, you should eat fish twice a week.

However, you should avoid farmed fish, because they are full of antibiotics and hormones. Like with humans, a fish's quality depends on what it eats, and it is often contaminated with harmful chemicals or even heavy metals.

You may be wondering: Does it have to be a fat ocean fish or will a fresh walleye do? In 1970, the Danish researchers Hans Olaf Bang and Jørn Dyerberg heard that the Inuit very seldom have cardiovascular disease. So the researchers flew over to investigate their diet. It consisted primarily of fatty whale and seal meat. Due to their climate, they didn't eat fruits and vegetables. Bang and Dyerberg concluded that it must be the fat. Had they looked at the actual frequency of their cardiovascular diseases, they would've noticed that it's just as high as in the Western world and that their average life expectancy was ten years shorter.

Nevertheless, a boom in omega-3 fish oil followed, even though it would soon be clear that it couldn't replace fish. The positive effect on blood vessels was never confirmed over all the years it was being recommended. This should remind us that it is always the whole food, not just an extract, that keeps us healthy and that our bodies have become accustomed to over thousands of years.

Very rarely is fish ever harmful to our digestive tract. Maybe you're thinking of the occasional bone that gets stuck in your throat. But you can be sure that never happens to those who chew their food well.

Meat

About a hundred years ago, we ate approximately 136 pounds of meat (red meat and poultry) per person every year. Today, that number is around 222 pounds a year—per person! This number can vary due to "meat scandals," like feeding pigs human waste, mad cow disease (BSE), rotten meat, horse meat, and other scandals. As soon as the media slows down its coverage, meat consumption rises again.

What does your meat consumption look like? The more red meat you eat, the higher your risk of developing colon cancer and cardiovascular disease. It's still not 100 percent clear why red meat leads to intestinal diseases more frequently. What is clear is that red meat contains a lot of L-carnitine, a chemical compound that is very significant for metabolizing energy in our cells. When we don't digest it properly, bacteria metabolize it in our intestines. This produces a toxic gas, trimethylamine, that causes cancer and partially causes arteriosclerosis.

Red meat is more difficult to digest than white meat, because it needs to be chewed more intensely. White meat's fibrous structure makes it more defenseless against stomach acids. So it's not the meat itself that make us sick, but rather inadequate chewing of the meat.

Malignant diseases arise almost exclusively in the two sections of the large intestine with the longest passage time. It doesn't have to be that way. If red meat arrives in the stomach optimally chewed, there would be nothing left after passing through the small intestine that could cause damage to the colon wall.

The quality of meat is of paramount importance, not only for your health, but also for the taste. Today's usual treatment of farm animals with antibiotics leads to deposits of medicine in their tissues, which is partially responsible for creating antibiotic-resistant germs. The taste also depends on what the animals are fed.

In conclusion, rules to follow when consuming red and white meat are to eat only good quality (organic, local meat), chew well, and treat yourself only two times a week!

Fruit

An apple a day keeps the doctor away. Why does it have to be an apple, of all fruits, to avoid going to the doctor? Because for a long time, apples were the only fruit that could be stored. But, in general, the saying is referring to fruit. Fruit reduces cancer and cardiovascular diseases when it's consumed at least three to five times a week.

A lot of people agree about fruit consumption, more than any other kind of food actually. The consensus is, "The more I eat, the better it is for my health"—and they are completely wrong!

Fruits contain a lot of fructose, which can only be absorbed in limited amounts. If you eat too much fruit, it ends up fermenting in your large intestine, which harms the bowel. One piece of fruit on a daily basis is sufficient.

For some tired intestines, one apple can already be too much. You'd notice it's too much by the excessive gas production. Cut back to half an apple, at least until the intestinal fitness program has improved your digestive performance, and then you can increase the portion again.

Drinks

As I mentioned earlier, it is incredibly difficult to specify the exact amount of fluids you should drink. It always depends on your physical activity and the liquid you lose through your skin, lungs, kidneys, and stool. It also depends on how much liquid you absorb from your food.

Look to the color of your urine as an indication: if it's almost transparent, with a touch of yellow, you're good to go.

Good drinks are water and unsweetened tea. They shouldn't be drunk during mealtime, but rather in between meals. Avoid juice and beverage-industry drinks; they contain too much fructose and sugar. The occasional drink is, of course, not going to hurt you.

And always remember, sufficient fluids are a prerequisite for an optimally functioning digestion.

Herbs and Spices

Don't hold back when it comes to herbs and spices, because then you'll need less salt. Most spices stimulate digestion and metabolism. The following spices are especially good at stimulating digestion: anise, mugwort, savory, chili, turmeric, tarragon, cloves, ginger, cardamom, cilantro, caraway, lovage, bay leaves, marjoram, horseradish, nutmeg, oregano, parsley, pepper, mint, rosemary, saffron, chives, mustard, and cinnamon.

Some herbs and spices have a soothing effect on digestion, such as fennel, sweet flag, lavender, and sage.

Smoothies

Smoothies are not just in vogue, but they're actually a good way to supplement your daily nourishment. They're nothing more than pureed fresh greens and fruits. Bananas and avocados are usually included in order to make the taste and consistency more pleasant.

In these chew-lazy times, the blender has taken away the tiresome crushing of greens. But this kitchen device doesn't produce saliva, which we need for good digestion. And smoothies have even more deficiencies.

If someone drinks too many smoothies—in other words, barely eats solid food—they're endangering their teeth, among other things. For us to have healthy teeth, nature provided us with a wonderful mechanism called chewing! It also helps us to salivate and feel full.

And similar to diets that completely omit animal products, smoothies are also missing vitamin B. So if you want to enjoy your smoothies, you'll have to supplement with B vitamins or eat foods that are rich in vitamin B. Fun and gross fact: monkeys primarily eat leaves, but they also enjoy eating their feces to fill up on vitamin B.

More than anything else, smoothies should contain greens and vegetables. Avoid adding fructose-rich fruits like apples and pears. The right amount is probably quite a bit less than most think a smoothie size should be: five fluid ounces. It's best to eat some nuts with each smoothie, so that you also produce enough essential saliva.

Coffee and Tea

Neither coffee nor tea counts as nourishment if you don't add sugar. Americans consume about 18.5 gallons of coffee per person per year. Black and green tea play a less important role in comparison, at only 10.3 gallons per person per year.

The stimulating effect of both drinks is ascribed to caffeine, as well as the effect on our circulation. People with low blood pressure can profit from drinking caffeine; for one or two hours, their blood pressure rises. Don't worry, though, if you have high blood pressure. Caffeine raises blood pressure only in those who don't drink it habitually.

In addition to the caffeine, coffee contains a mixture of over a thousand different chemicals, mostly roasted substances, which are responsible for the effect coffee has on the digestive tract. This may vary substantially depending on the kind of coffee bean and its preparation. These roasted substances stimulate the production of digestive secretions in the stomach and small intestine, as well as bile flow. For some, the declining elasticity in the lower part of the esophagus is the cause of heartburn. Upon sensing irritation in the upper part of the digestive tract, the large intestine reacts with stimulated peristalsis, facilitating the walk to the toilet. For many this is a welcome side effect, but for people with a hypersensitive digestive tract, sheer horror. The excessive consumption of coffee, thus sensory overload, can reverse all the welcome effects. Digestive help then becomes constipation, which is another reason for moderate consumption.

Headaches from caffeine withdrawal can also be attributed to the effect caffeine has on our blood vessels. Some people—and it's genetically determined—only break down caffeine in a limited way. Drinking it leads to an unintentional overdose, which then causes a tightening of the vessels that can cause a heart attack. It's another reason to enjoy it in moderation.

In the case of green tea especially, the antioxidant effects reduce the risk of colon cancer if consumed in large quantities. Unfortunately, coffee doesn't have the same effect because of the roasting process.

Enjoy a cup of coffee or tea! And if you suddenly no longer tolerate it, take a break or change brands or preparation.

Carbohydrates

Carbohydrates, also called *saccharides*, are sugars and starches. We differentiate between monosaccharides (one sugar molecule), disaccharides (two sugar molecules), and polysaccharides, which include starches (about two hundred sugar molecules).

For us, the most important carbohydrate—in other words the most important supplier of energy—is a monosaccharide called *glucose.*

For decades, the food industry considered bread and noodles, both of which contain a lot of starch, the most essential food for us. In the familiar nutrition pyramid, carbohydrates took up the most room. For years, people lived off of bread, noodles, and a ton of sugar. The average body weight rose from year to year, diabetes became widespread, and it was more and more difficult for the food industry to find support from the medical world for their favorite food products.

Anyone would naturally come to the conclusion that carbohydrates stuck us with many of our lifestyle diseases. But again, it depends on the amount we consume. As mentioned earlier, we eat half the amount of bread we ate one hundred years ago, while we eat twice the sugar. Therefore, we should be especially careful with sugar consumption.

If you're not satisfied with your weight, avoid sugar, don't eat more than a slice of bread per day, and consume pasta no more than twice a week.

For digestion, extremely starchy foods (rice, potatoes, grains, and corn) are problematic if they're not chewed really well. There is an enzyme in the saliva (amylase) that starts breaking down starches in the mouth, and if this doesn't happen, more undigested starches reach the large intestine, where bacteria happily throw themselves at the meal. Once again, the bacterial toxin and gas production is triggered.

Mediterranean Diet

The Mediterranean diet is the healthiest form of nutrition, according to most studies. Along with cultural and country-specific differences, this diet reflects the way northern Mediterranean countries ate until the middle of the twentieth century. The way most of their citizens eat today has nothing to do with a Mediterranean diet.

Numerous studies have shown that this diet can prevent cardiovascular disease as well as depression, breast cancer, colon cancer, diabetes, obesity, asthma, impotency, and difficulty concentrating.

Naturally, we have to ask ourselves what a Mediterranean diet is exactly and what price we would have to pay if we followed it. It's a delicious mix of vegetables, fruits, nuts, fish, and olive oil, with a small portion of meat, dairy products, and grains. The price for many is having to reduce sugar, meat, grains, and dairy products, but the reward is a healthy life thanks to a delicious variety of produce.

Dairy Products

Even if cow milk is meant for calves and not us, it is a part of our diet, along with all the other dairy products. The problem is how much of our diet it has become. It wasn't so long ago that we consumed dairy products irregularly and in small amounts.

Today, we often add milk to our coffee and cereal, or yogurt to our granola and smoothies. Then, throughout the day, we enjoy eating cheese on our bread, sour cream on our nachos, and, between meals, a strawberry yogurt that is full of sugar and usually doesn't even contain real fruit. That is way too much!

The right quantity would be one cup of yogurt with fresh fruit and no sugar, *or* a little milk, *or* a dab of sour cream, *or* a small piece of cheese. You shouldn't eat dairy products daily, and if you do, then only in small amounts.

Remember that milk protein may be a trigger for inflammatory skin disorders like acne and eczema. And if you have regular flatulence after drinking a cappuccino, you can bet you belong to the 25 percent of the United States population that cannot digest lactose.

When buying dairy products, make sure they come from animals that are pasture raised and grass fed. You want unprocessed dairy. Raw milk, organic yogurt, and raw-milk cheese will put you on the right path.

Cereal, Granola, and Muesli

Health-conscious people are used to eating granola for breakfast. The variety in grocery stores can be overwhelming . . . and tempting. Granola is indeed a wonderful opportunity for us to eat nuts, fruits, seeds, and maybe a few cornflakes, and to start the day off right.

Unfortunately, there are other issues with it besides the critical amount of milk consumption. Many of the granola brands for sale are difficult to digest because they're not prepared correctly. For example, some of them contain ingredients that need to be cooked or soaked for a while, like oats and dried fruit, while others have ingredients that turn to a slimy mush if you cook or soak them too long. Have you ever tried cooking cornflakes?

Clearly, it's better not to cook or soak them. But then you'd need forty-five minutes every morning to chew everything properly. As long as you do, granola is fine for digestion.

Instead of granola, the British love porridge (oatmeal). It's a very easily digestible breakfast option that doesn't need milk or juice to boot. It's eaten warm and can be ground, crushed, steel cut, or rolled. You can prepare it with apples and raisins, or add ingredients after cooking, such as bananas, cherries, blueberries, maple syrup, nuts, or cinnamon.

But if you can't do without your granola or muesli in the morning, there's an easy solution: Make it yourself. Then you can select the best ingredients for your digestion. You simply mix it all together in a large glass jar, cover it, shake it all up, and voila! Breakfast is served perfectly every time. Of course, you'll still need to chew well, but at least you'll avoid the flatulence!

Artificial Sweeteners

Now, here is one very serious warning: Stay away from artificial sweeteners! They are supposed to replace sugar, but their sweetness actually surpasses it. So if you're trying to break the habit of eating sugar, these sweeteners are useless.

The first artificial sweeteners were introduced at the end of the nineteenth century, and only people with diabetes who had a prescription could purchase them at a pharmacy.

Research done by Jotham Suez and his colleagues from the Weizmann Institute of Science in Israel confirmed the suspicion that many diabetologists had been considering for a long time—artificial sweeteners are a trigger for diabetes. In animal testing, these sweeteners changed the intestinal flora. It started working hard to produce sugar out of all the remains and then make it available for the body. As a result, the mice started having metabolic disorders.

A large European study on nutrition from 2015 showed that a daily glass of soda increases the risk of diabetes by 21 percent, regardless of whether it contains sugar or artificial sweetener.

The question of whether or not artificial sweeteners cause cancer has been debated for several years. Until now, a slightly higher risk of bladder cancer has been confirmed. However, reliable statements can only be made when the sweetener in question has been on the market for a very long time, which is not the case for many artificial sweeteners.

Stevia, a plant that can be 450 times sweeter than sugar depending on the dosage, is also considered an artificial sweetener. The "sweet leaf" comes from South America and is used in small amounts by the indigenous population to sweeten their food.

Research from 1982 proving that stevia is cancer causing prevented it from reaching the market for many decades. It wasn't until 2011 that stevia was allowed to be sold in Europe. "Stevia is natural," claimed the most important sales argument. But consider poison oak—just because something is natural, that doesn't automatically mean it's nontoxic.

Considering the effects they have on the intestines and metabolism, I'd like to repeat one more time that you should avoid consuming non-nutritive sweeteners. If you want to sweeten something, use small amounts of natural sweeteners, such as cane juice, muscovado cane sugar, honey, agave syrup, or something similar.

A Vegan Diet

People who don't consume or use any animal products or byproducts are usually not doing it for their health, but rather for ideological reasons. In the history of mankind, animal-derived foods were always around, even if we used to eat less of them. For vegans, something is missing that has been on the menu for thousands of years.

There are still not enough studies done on this kind of diet to be able to make a definitive assessment about the related health aspects, but vegans do tend to have a higher level of homocysteine in the blood. Homocysteine is a natural amino acid found in the body. If it is not broken down sufficiently, it can lead to blood vessel damage and dementia in the elderly. We need vitamin B_{12} to break homocysteine down, and vegans don't consume sufficient amounts of it. Taking B_{12} supplements can help lower the homocysteine in the blood; however, it's still being debated if it has any real clinical use.

It is possible that other not-yet-proven substances are missing in a vegan diet. Therefore, if you follow a vegan diet, be sure to consult the latest scientific developments regularly. This way, you'll be able to react quickly if any new health disadvantages are discovered.

Vegetarian Diet

A vegetarian doesn't eat any food products that contain dead animal. Unlike a vegan diet, vegetarians eat protein and vitamin-rich eggs and, often, too many dairy products.

It is undisputed that vegetarians lead healthier lives! They have fewer instances of high blood pressure, heart attacks, diabetes, cancer, and rheumatism. They live even longer if they also avoid alcohol, tobacco, sugar, and too many dairy products.

The intestines of a vegetarian are grateful. Eating more fibrous vegetables aids intestinal peristalsis, which then lowers the occurrence of diverticula and colon cancer.

Nevertheless, as is the case in most diets, the quantity can be a problem (along with the chewing). You should be prudent when it comes to eating healthy but difficult-to-digest crudités. You should eat only as much as your intestines can handle. Again, if you feel gassy after eating a lot of vegetables, slow down.

Besides raw vegetables, vegetarians' consumption of dairy products can cause them some trouble. Research in Europe and Asia shows interesting differences. European vegetarians have softer bones and develop cancer (not colon cancer) just as often as meat eaters do. This is not the case in Asia, where they barely consume any dairy products at all.

Sugar

Above, I talked about artificial sweeteners, and now on to our favorite subject—sugar. At the end of the nineteenth century, sugar consumption was at thirty pounds per person, and one hundred years later, it was at eighty-eight pounds per person. Even if these numbers haven't changed much from then until today, we shouldn't forget about all the new suppliers of sugars. Like artificial sweeteners, glucose and fructose are found everywhere. The food industry is well aware of this delicious flavoring component. The average American consumes sixty-six pounds of added sugar every year.

As I said earlier, sugar is poison, and the damage it causes is as wide-ranging as alcohol and cigarettes. Sugar contributes to cardiovascular as well as metabolic diseases. And thanks to our parents' constant reminder, we'll never forget: sugar rots your teeth.

We need to remember that the food industry often adds sugar to make tasteless food with low nutritional value tasty. In this case, it's hard to tell if our health is damaged by the sugar or by the low-grade food product.

If consumed in large amounts, sugar alters the intestinal flora, and you already know what the results are. But what exactly is a "large amount"?

The answer to this question is well documented. If you were to drink a liter (a quart) of any industrially manufactured beverage every day to quench your thirst, you would be consuming about 80 pounds of sugar annually. In order to reach this amount of sugar eating dark chocolate, you would have to consume about 220 pounds. That means 4 pounds of chocolate per week!

But a daily quart of soda isn't even close to the total amount of sugar some of us consume. We have to add the sugar from flavored yogurt, chocolate, pastries, and all the other snacks we eat and don't realize contain sugar until we read the finely printed ingredients on the back.

So, how much is a healthy amount of sugar? The American Heart Association states that men should eat no more than nine teaspoons (thirty-eight grams) of added sugar a day and for women, no more than six teaspoons (twenty-five grams) of added sugar a day. Basically, you want to keep your sugar consumption to a minimum. Now, it's impractical to go around measuring the sugar content in every item; it would be exhausting and even impossible to do this if, say, you were enjoying a homemade desert. So you can easily limit sugar in your diet by following these simple rules: Avoid all sweetened beverages, whether artificially or naturally sweetened. That even includes 100 percent natural juice. Don't eat mass-produced flavored yogurt since it's chock-full of added and natural sugar. And of course, try to avoid processed foods when you can. Lastly, don't eat anything sweet between meals, in order to give your digestive tract, and especially your pancreas, a break.

Don't worry—you can still enjoy your dessert or that piece of chocolate with your coffee after a meal. In these quantities, sugar isn't poisonous, but rather a joy, a treat. The quantity is what makes it toxic. So remember to avoid eating sugary foods and drinks between meals. No snacking on sweets!

Below is a look into how much adults consume in a year—past and present:

Milk consumption per person in 1860	0 gallons
Milk consumption per person in 2017	23 gallons
Meat consumption per person in 1909	136 pounds
Meat consumption per person in 2018	222 pounds
Bread consumption per person in 1850	550 pounds
Bread consumption per person in 2016	122 pounds
Sugar consumption per person in 1700	4 pounds
Sugar consumption per person in 1800	18 pounds
Sugar consumption per person in 2017	66 pounds
Fiber consumption per person in 1850	62 pounds
Fiber consumption per person in 2017	13 pounds

SAVE THE BEST FOR LAST

It's not at all difficult to influence your overall health by caring for your intestines. The knowledge you've now gained about the digestive process will help you for a lifetime. Maybe you're one of the lucky few who only needs to change a few small details. If you are currently doing everything wrong regarding your intestinal health, don't try to change too much at once. Chew training requires a certain amount of perseverance and is definitely one of the more difficult things to change. You won't be able to master it overnight, but you'll improve every week. Not eating too much at dinner, as well as avoiding snacks, is a question of discipline. If it doesn't work right away, don't worry. People are creatures of habit. After a few weeks without snacking, you'll be asking yourself how you were ever capable of constantly eating between meals.

At least once a year, try to make it through ten days of an intestinal fitness program. This will help you balance out some of the errors you can't avoid committing during the year.

Basically, you can eat almost anything you want as long as you figure out the right quantity. As soon as your bowel is healthy again, it will let you know what it needs.

I wrote this book to fill a gap of missing knowledge I noticed in thousands of my patients and to show you an easy way to improve your overall health. I wish you the best of luck on your journey!

Acknowledgments

Without your encouragement, dear Charles, this book wouldn't exist. Thank you so much! I'd like to thank my friends Robert and Nils for always being there for me when I needed direction and understanding.

Jürgen, Fredy, Christine, Lothar, and my sister Astrid: thank you for your time and valuable ideas!

Thanks a lot, Justine, for covering for me during my writing weeks and conjuring up important illustrations at the last minute.

I'd also like to thank my German publishers, Mr. Strasser and Ms. Olzog, for believing in me. And, Ms. Buergel-Goodwin, I thank you for reviewing my manuscript, along with all the employees at the publishing house who invested their time and energy in my book.

Thanks to all of my patients—your desire to read everything I've taught you during conversations and seminars pushed me to keep writing.

I'm grateful to all the employees at the medical clinic, F. X. Mayr Zentrum Bodensee, for showing me that our patients felt just as comfortable and healthy without me while I wrote this book.

Selected Bibliography and Resources

This is a list of books and journal articles that have been used in the research for this book. This bibliography is by no means a complete record of all the works and sources I have consulted. It indicates the substance and range of reading upon which I have formed my ideas, and I intend it to serve as a convenience for those who wish to further pursue the study of intestinal health.

PART 1. A Travel Guide to Your Digestive Tract

Bollinger, R. Randal, Andrew S. Barbas, Errol L. Bush, Shu S. Lin, and William Parker. "Biofilms in the Large Bowel Suggest an Apparent Function of the Human Vermiform Appendix." *Journal of Theoretical Biology* 249, no. 4 (December 2007): 826–831. https://www.ncbi.nlm.nih.gov/pubmed/17936308.

Fletcher, Horace. *Fletcherism: What It Is; or, How I Became Young at Sixty*. Miami, Florida: HardPress Publishing, 2013.

Hirano, Yoshiyuki and Minoru Onozuka. "Chewing and Cognitive Function." *Brain and Nerve* 66, no. 1 (January 2014): 25–32. https://www.ncbi.nlm.nih.gov/pubmed/24371128.

Kokkinos, Alexander, Carel W. le Roux, Kleopatra Alexiadou, Nicholas Tentolouris, Royce P. Vincent, Despoina Kyriaki, Despoina Perrea,

Mohammad A. Ghatei, Stephen R. Bloom, and Nicholas Katsilambros. "Eating Slowly Increases the Postprandial Response of the Anorexigenic Gut Hormones, Peptide YY and Glucagon-Like Peptide-1," *Journal of Clinical Endocrinology & Metabolism* 95, no. 1 (January 2010): 333–337. https://www.ncbi.nlm.nih.gov /pubmed/19875483.

Rauch, Erich and Florian Rauch. *Health through Inner Body Cleansing: The Famous F. X Mayr Intestinal Therapy from Europe*, 7th Edition. New York: Thieme Publishers, 2016.

Sikirov, D. "Comparison of Straining During Defecation in Three Positions: Results and Implications for Human Health," *Digestive Diseases and Sciences* 48, no. 7 (July 2003): 1201–1205. https://www.ncbi .nlm.nih.gov/pubmed/12870773.

Smit, Hendrik Jan, E. Katherine Kemsley, Henri S. Tapp, and C. Jeya K. Henry. "Does Prolonged Chewing Reduce Food Intake? Fletcherism Revisited," *Appetite*. 57, no. 1 (August 2011): 295–298. https:// www.ncbi.nlm.nih.gov/pubmed/21316411.

Weizman, Adam V. and Geoffrey C. Nguyen. "Diverticular Disease: Epidemiology and Management," *Canadian Journal of Gastroenterology* 25, no. 7 (July 2011): 385-389. https://www.ncbi.nlm.nih.gov /pubmed/21876861.

PART 2. On a Wayward Path

Campbell, T. Collin and Thomas M. Campbell II. *The China Study: The Most Comprehensive Study of Nutrition Ever Conducted and the Startling Implications for Diet, Weight Loss and Long-Term Health*. Dallas, Texas: Benbella Books, 2005.

Catassi, Carlo, Julio C. Bai, Bruno Bonaz, Gerd Bouma, Antonio Calabrò, Antonio Carroccio, Gemma Castillejo, et al. "Non-Celiac Gluten Sensitivity: The New Frontier of Gluten Related Disorders," *Nutrients* 4, no. 10 (September 2013): 3839–3853. https://www.ncbi.nlm.nih .gov/pmc/articles/PMC3820047/.

Cummings, J. H. and G. T. Macfarlane. "The Control and Consequences of Bacterial Fermentation in the Human Colon," *Journal of Applied Microbiology* 70, no. 6 (June 1991): 443–459. https://www.ncbi .nlm.nih.gov/pubmed/1938669.

Drago, Sandro, Ramzi El Asmar, Mariarosaria Di Pierro, Maria Grazia Clemente, Amit Tripathi, Anna Sapone, Manjusha Thakar, et al. "Gliadin, Zonulin and Gut Permeability: Effects on Celiac and Non-Celiac Intestinal Mucosa and Intestinal Cell Lines," *Scandinavian Journal of Gastroenterology* 41, no. 4 (April 2006): 408–419. https:// www.tandfonline.com/doi/abs/10.1080/00365520500235334.

Kellogg, J. H. *Autointoxication; or, Intestinal Toxemia*. London: Forgotten Books, 2017.

Koeth, Robert A., Zeneng Wang, Bruce S. Levison, Jennifer A. Buffa, Elin Org, Brendan T. Sheehy, Earl B. Britt, et al. "Intestinal Microbiota Metabolism of L-Carnitine, a Nutrient in Red Meat, Promotes Atherosclerosis," *Nature Medicine* 19, no. 5 (May 2013): 576–585. https://www.ncbi.nlm.nih.gov/pmc/articles/PMC3650111/.

Lammers, Karen M., Ruliang Lu, Julie Brownley, Bao Lu, Craig Gerard, Karen Thomas, Prasad Rallabhandi, et al. "Gliadin Induces an Increase in Intestinal Permeability and Zonulin Release by Binding to the Chemokine Receptor CXCR3," *Gastroenterology* 135, no.1 (July 2008): 194–204. https://www.ncbi.nlm.nih.gov/pmc/articles /PMC2653457/.

Mayer, Emeran A. "Gut feelings: The Emerging Biology of Gut–Brain Communication," *Nature Reviews Neuroscience* 12, no. 8 (July 2011): 453–466. https://www.nature.com/articles/nrn3071.

Michaëlsson, Karl, Alicja Wolk, Sophie Langenskiöld, Samar Basu, Eva Warensjö Lemming, Håkan Melhus, and Liisa Byberg. "Milk Intake and Risk of Mortality and Fractures in Women and Men: Cohort Studies," *British Medical Journal* 349 (October 2014): 6015. https://www.ncbi.nlm.nih.gov/pubmed/25352269.

Smith, Caroline, Heather Hancock, Jane Blake-Mortimer, and Kerena Eckert. "A Randomised Comparative Trial of Yoga and Relaxation to Reduce Stress and Anxiety," *Complementary Therapies in Medicine* 15, no. 2 (June 2007): 77–83. https://www.sciencedirect.com/science/article/pii/S0965229906000434.

Tang, W. H. Wilson, Zeneng Wang, Bruce S. Levison, Robert A. Koeth, Earl B. Britt, Xiaoming Fu, Yuping Wu, and Stanley Hazen. "Intestinal Microbial Metabolism of Phosphatidylcholine and Cardiovascular Risk," *New England Journal of Medicine* 368, no. 17 (April 2013): 1575–1584. https://www.nejm.org/doi/10.1056/NEJMoa1109400.

Tatar, Gonca, Rengin Elsurer, Halis Simsek, Yasemin H. Balaban, Osman I. Ozcebe, and Yahya Buyukasik. "Screening of Tissue Transglutaminase Antibody in Healthy Blood Donors for Celiac Disease Screening in the Turkish Population," *Digestive Diseases and Science* 49, no. 9 (2004): 1479–1484. https://www.ncbi.nlm.nih.gov/pubmed/15481323.

PART 3. On the Right Track

Bäckhed, Fredrik. "Meat-Metabolizing Bacteria in Atherosclerosis," *Nature Medicine* 19 (May 2013): 533–534. https://www.nature.com/articles/nm.3178.

Bae, Sajin, Cornelia M. Ulrich, Marian L. Neuhouser, Olga Malysheva, Lynn B. Bailey, Liren Xiao, Elissa C. Brown, et al. "Plasma Choline Metabolites and Colorectal Cancer Risk in the Women's Health Initiative Observational Study," *Cancer Research* 74, no. 24 (December 2014): 7442-7452. http://cancerres.aacrjournals.org/content/74/24/7442.

Blaser, Martin J. *Missing Microbes: How the Overuse of Antibiotics Is Fueling Our Modern Plagues.* New York: Picador-Macmillan, 2015.

Brown, Rebecca J. and Kristina I. Rother. "Non-Nutritive Sweeteners and Their Role in the Gastrointestinal Tract," *Journal of Clinical Endocrinology and Metabolism* 97, no. 8 (August 2012): 2597–2605. https://academic.oup.com/jcem/article/97/8/2597/2823224.

Fagherazzi, Guy, Alice Vilier, Daniela Saes Sartorelli, Martin Lajous, Beverely Balkau, and Françoise Clavel-Chapelon. "Consumption of Artificially and Sugar-Sweetened Beverages and Incident Type 2 Diabetes in the Etude Epidémiologique auprès Des Femmes de la Mutuelle Générale de l'Education Nationale—European Prospective Investigation into Cancer and Nutrition Cohort," *American Journal of Clinical Nutrition* 97, no. 3 (January 2013) 517–523. https://academic.oup.com/ajcn/article/97/3/517/4571511.

Fodor, J. George, Eftyhia Helis, Narges Yazdekhasti, and Branislav Vohnout. "'Fishing' for the Origins of the 'Eskimos and Heart Disease' Story: Facts or Wishful Thinking?," *Canadian Journal of Cardiology* 30, no. 8 (April 2014): 864–868. https://www.onlinecjc .ca/article/S0828-282X(14)00237-2/fulltext.

Kwok, Chun Shing, Saadia Umar, Phyo K. Myint, Mamas A. Mamas, and Yoon K. Loke. "Vegetarian Diet, Seventh Day Adventists and Risk of Cardiovascular Mortality: A Systematic Review and Meta-Aanalysis," *International Journal of Cardiology* 176, no. 3 (October 2014): 680– 686. https://www.internationaljournalofcardiology.com/article /S0167-5273(14)01290-X/fulltext.

Lee, C. and Valter D. Longo. "Fasting Vs Dietary Restriction in Cellu- lar Protection and Cancer Treatment: From Model Organisms to Patients," *Oncogene* 30, no. 30 (July 2011): 3305–3316. https:// www.nature.com/articles/onc201191.

Longo, Valter D. and Luigi Fontana. "Calorie Restriction and Cancer Prevention: Metabolic and Molecular Mechanisms," *Trends in Phar- macological Sciences* 31, no. 2 (January 2010): 89–98. https://www .ncbi.nlm.nih.gov/pubmed/20097433.

Manz, F. "Hydration and Disease," *Journal of the American College of Nutri- tion* 26, no. 5 Suppl (October 2007): 535S–541S. https://www.ncbi .nlm.nih.gov/pubmed/17921462.

Matt, Katja, Katharina Burger, Daniel Gebhard, and Jörg Bergemann. "Influence of Calorie Reduction on DNA Repair Capacity of Human Peripheral Blood Mononuclear Cells," *Mechanisms of Ageing and Development* 154 (March 2016): 24-29. https://www.sciencedirect .com/science/article/pii/S0047637416300136.

McCay, C. M. "Effect of Restricted Feeding upon Aging and Chronic Diseases in Rats and Dogs," *American Journal of Public Health* 37, no. 5 (May 1947): 521-528. https://www.ncbi.nlm.nih.gov/pmc /articles/PMC1623629/.

Rizos, Evangelos C., Evangelia E. Ntzani, Effychia Bika, Michael S. Kostapanos, and Moses S. Elisaf. "Association Between Omega-3 Fatty Acid Supplementation and Risk of Major Cardiovascular Disease Events: A Systematic Review and Meta-Analysis," *Jama* 308, no. 10 (September 2012): 1024–1033. https://jamanetwork.com /journals/jama/article-abstract/1357266.

Soffritti, Morando, Michela Padovani, Eva Tibaldi, Laura Falcioni, Fabiana Manservisi, and Fiorella Belpoggi. "The Carcinogenic Effects of Aspartame: The Urgent Need for Regulatory Re-evaluation," *American Journal of Industrial Medicine* 57, no. 4 (January 2014): 383–397. https://onlinelibrary.wiley.com/doi/abs/10.1002/ajim.22296.

Suez, Jotham, Tal Korem, David Zeevi, Gili Zilberman-Schapira, Christoph A. Thaiss, Ori Maza, David Israeli, et al. "Artificial Sweeteners Induce Glucose Intolerance by Altering the Gut Microbiota," *Nature* 514, no. 7521 (October 2014): 181–186. https://www.nature.com /articles/nature13793.

Wang, Xia, Yingying Ouyang, Jun Liu, Minmin Zhu, Gang Zhao, Wei Bao, and Frank B. Hu. "Fruit and Vegetable Consumption and Mortality from All Causes, Cardiovascular Disease, and Cancer: Systematic Review and Dose-Response Meta-Analysis of Prospective Cohort Studies," *British Medical Journal* 349 (July 2014): g4490. https://www.ncbi.nlm.nih.gov/pmc/articles/PMC4115152/.

Widmer, R. Jay, Andreas J. Flammer, Lilach O. Lerman, and Amir Lerman. "The Mediterranean Diet, Its Components, and Cardiovascular Disease," *American Journal of Medicine* 128, no. 3 (October

2014): 229–238. https://www.ncbi.nlm.nih.gov/pmc/articles/PMC 4339461/.

Yudkin, John. *Pure, White and Deadly: How Sugar Is Killing Us and What We Can Do to Stop It*. New York: Penguin Books, 2013.

ADDITIONAL RESOURCES

If you decide to seek additional professional assistance to get your gut back in shape, I have a few recommendations (all websites can be viewed in English).

The clinic I work out of is the F. X. Mayr Bodensee Center in Überlingen/Hödingen, where you'll be treated by many wonderful trained specialists and doctors while relaxing in an idyllic lake retreat setting with peaceful gardens and beautiful accommodations.

F. X. Mayr Zentrum Bodensee
Brunnenstraße 30a
88662 Überlingen
www.fxmayr.eu
info@fxmayr.eu

In the United States, I recommend Dr. Kevin Alan and Dr. Arina Cadariu. These two physicians are currently the only two practicing Mayr Medicine within the states.

Kevin Alen, MD
63 Port Royal Dr.
Palm Coast, Florida 32164
Phone: 904-824-9439
Email: kevin.alen@gmail.com

Arina Cadariu, MD MPH
Assistant Clinical Professor of Medicine
Internal Medicine Attending
Yale School of Medicine
233 Mansfield Grove Road Unit 503
East Haven, CT 06512
Cell Phone: 203-214-4617
Email: cadariu@hotmail.com
arcadariu@aya.yale.edu

Below is the International Society of Mayr Physicians website, where you can find specialized centers all over the world. You are also able to get special Mayr's training in English, but this is not a treatment center.

Internationale Gesellschaft der Mayr-Ärzte
Kochholzweg 153
A-6072 Lans
www.fxmayr.com
office@fxmayr.com

Index